487 Really Cool Tips for Kids with Diabetes

Spike Nasmyth Loy and Bo Nasmyth Loy

American Diabetes Association®
Cure • Care • Commitment®

Director, Book Publishing, John Fedor; *Associate Director, Consumer Books,* Sherrye Landrum; *Editors,* Abe Ogden and Sherrye Landrum; *Associate Director, Book Production,* Peggy M. Rote; *Composition*, Circle Graphics, Inc.; *Cover Design,* Koncept Inc.; *Printer,* Worzalla

Printed in the United States of America
1 3 5 7 9 10 8 6 4 2

The suggestions and information contained in this publication are generally consistent with the *Clinical Practice Recommendations* and other policies of the American Diabetes Association, but they do not represent the policy or position of the Association or any of its boards or committees. Reasonable steps have been taken to ensure the accuracy of the information presented. However, the American Diabetes Association cannot ensure the safety or efficacy of any product or service described in this publication. Individuals are advised to consult a physician or other appropriate health care professional before undertaking any diet or exercise program or taking any medication referred to in this publication. Professionals must use and apply their own professional judgment, experience, and training and should not rely solely on the information contained in this publication before prescribing any diet, exercise, or medication. The American Diabetes Association—its officers, directors, employees, volunteers, and members—assumes no responsibility or liability for personal or other injury, loss, or damage that may result from the suggestions or information in this publication.

∞ The paper in this publication meets the requirements of the ANSI Standard Z39.48-1992 (permanence of paper).

ADA titles may be purchased for business or promotional use or for special sales. To purchase this book in large quantities, or for custom editions of this book with your logo, contact Lee Romano Sequeira, Special Sales & Promotions, at the address below, or at LRomano@diabetes.org or 703-299-2046.

American Diabetes Association
1701 North Beauregard Street
Alexandria, Virginia 22311

Library of Congress Cataloging-in-Publication Data

Loy, Bo Nasmyth, 1982-
487 really cool tips for kids / Bo Nasmyth Loy, Spike Nasmyth Loy.
p. cm.
Includes index.
ISBN 1-58040-191-0 (pbk. : alk. paper)
1. Diabetes in children—Juvenile literature. 2. Diabetes in adolescence—Juvenile literature. I. Title:Four hundred eighty-seven really cool tips for kids. II. Loy, Spike Nasmyth, 1980- III. Title.

RJ420.D5L693 2004
618.92'462—dc22

2004051819

Contents

Foreword

Tips for Kids is the sequel to Spike and Bo Loy's previous book *Getting a Grip on Diabetes.* It also is the third contribution of the Loy family in their quest to share their lives and diabetes experiences with other families who are traveling a similar road. I am honored to write the foreword to Spike and Bo's new book, as I was to write the foreword for their mother Virginia's book, *Real Life Parenting*, written specifically for other parents of children with diabetes.

In *Tips for Kids*, Spike and Bo expand on *Getting a Grip* by building a network of youth with diabetes, and obtaining life stories and diabetes coping strategies from many of their peers. I have witnessed firsthand the ability of Bo and Spike to connect with and serve as role models for other young people dealing with diabetes. In this current book, many of these children now get to have their voices heard, and thereby serve as teachers and mentors for other children. Thus, the circle grows and the interconnections of community are expanded. This is just one of the many gifts of this book.

Despite all the technological advances we have seen in diabetes care in recent years, the need for human connection still cries out. The journey through life with diabetes is not easy, and has the potential to be a lonely one. One of the first things I tell any child who has just developed diabetes is to share the news. Tell family, friends, and teachers of your experiences. A major theme of *Tips for Kids* is this message to kids with diabetes: Tell everyone your story! Share your life! Besides serving your practical needs, how will the basketball coach know you need juice if you haven't told him what you look like when you have a low sugar? This enables you to own this new aspect of your identity, to gather pride from educating others and reducing stereotypes. Remember that no matter how much knowledge a doctor or diabetes educator may have about diabetes, the real "experts" are you—the people who live, day in and day out, with diabetes.

In this book, we hear from the experts. And they speak with golden tongues and pearls of wisdom far beyond their years. Their words will be helpful to many people, on many levels. I hope physicians and health professionals will pick up this book and use it to gain insight into the realities of their patients' lives. The book is for parents as well, to know that their children share experiences and challenges with other children—and perhaps to gain a bit more understanding and information to help guide their own child through his or her life with diabetes. And lastly, and of course most importantly, it is for the children. You need to know that you are the experts on your lives, and that what you have to say is important and needed. Acknowledging this fact is one of the most important gifts we can give our children.

With warm regards,
Marc J. Weigensberg, MD

Acknowledgments

Thanks!

We had a great time gathering tips for this book. We met some amazing kids and learned so much from all of the stories we heard. So first and foremost, we want to say a gigantic "Thanks!" to the more than 100 kids who shared their tips and their stories with us. You guys wrote this thing!

We want to especially thank everyone at PADRE (Pediatric Adolescent Diabetes Research and Education) for helping so much. It's been great hanging out with such a fun bunch. Thank you Jackie, Bryan, Christine, A. J., and all the kids at PADRE.

Our mother would never forgive us if we neglected to thank all of the mothers and fathers who shared tips with us, too. Thank you for the stories and the emails and for taking care of your kids with diabetes so well. To all of you who read over our rough, rough drafts of this book an extra thanks for your wonderful suggestions. A special thanks to our Aunt Gebo for her impeccable editing, to Lyra Halprin for her comments, Jana Headman for making copious copies, and to Renea Clay for her computer work.

Thank you to Dr. Marc Weigensberg, everyone's favorite endocrinologist, for all of his additions and for being a friend and mentor.

Sherrye and Abe at the American Diabetes Association have been putting in overtime and deserve a big thanks for getting this book printed. Thanks for all the hard work.

Thanks to Susan Sheridan of Susan Sheridan Photography, who was kind enough to let us use a lot of her fine photos of kids (we should say, contributors) in this book.

A special thanks to kids who contributed stories about whole chunks of their lives so other kids could figure out diabetes a little faster: Derrick Crowe, the Gadget Kid; Julia Halprin Jackson, camp counselor and rower; Mary Costello for her work on traveling and water polo; Blair Ryan for her very detailed insight on competitive running; Jessica Stogsdill for riding dirt bikes and telling us about it; Jennifer Ogden for her tips on surgery—and dating; Jenna Rinaldi for tackling 'girl stuff'; Brooks Kincaid and Rory Tarbox for talking about college life and sports; enthusiastic Hanna Smith for sharing how-to-handle softball and basketball; Mollie Meggs in Georgia, for sharing how to be organized when competing in cheer and dance; Kelly Hrubeniuk, the backpacker; Rollie Berry for sharing his pocket full of glucagon goo while snorkeling; Chris and Cory Graham for sharing brother stuff; and a special thanks to our favorite princess, Laura Valine.

What kind of sons would we be if we didn't thank Mom? The kind that aren't getting any more breakfasts, that's what kind! Mom, thank you so much for your hard work on this book and for letting us leave all the messy work to you. But thanks mostly for taking such good care of us and for being, quite honestly, the best mom any kid (especially a kid with diabetes) could ask for.

Introduction

Bo: Spike and I had a really neat childhood growing up on a ranch. We included our friends in everything we did and let everybody know about our diabetes. One of the things we realized over the years is that sharing diabetes strengthened our family and our community.

From idyllic summers of swimming, running through the hills, and endless moto-cross track building, enduring friendships grew. Those friendships were strengthened when, on occasion, Spike or I needed a little help. We were diagnosed with insulin-dependent diabetes at ages 7 and 6, and there were a lot of times when our friends helped us deal with it. A typical incident occurred when I was out surfing with my friends Erik and Ryan. I crashed while I was fairly far out in the water. My blood sugar levels dropped fast. Feeling weak, I sort of collapsed on my board. Eric was right there. He grabbed the nose of my board, paddled us in, and fed me candy and Coke until I felt better.

When diabetes came to our family, we got busy. We began raising a special breed of pigs called Large Whites for islet cell research. One day a week, we would stay home from school and help our mother surgically remove the pancreas of a pig for transplant research. It was a community effort. Our neighbors

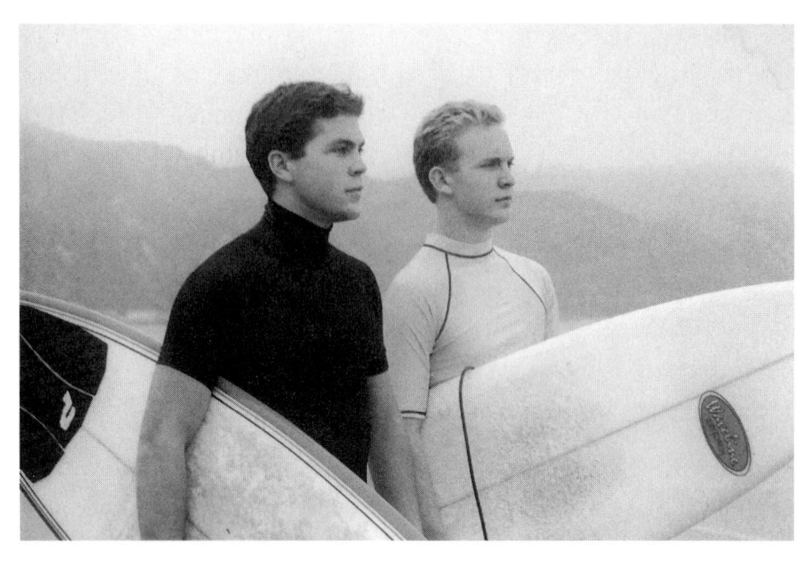

Spike Bo

Gan, Chris, Phil, Margaret, and Mandy were always there when the lab needed a pancreas. In the beginning my job was to time how long it took to extract the pancreas and put it on ice in a cooler filled with a digestive enzyme solution. Later I talked Mom into giving me a surgical gown and gloves and actually helped with removing the organs. It was incredibly rewarding to participate in the search for a cure for diabetes.

As the little boy with the watch timing the surgery, I didn't realize how much our community was involved in our efforts. When I got older and started to think about it, I realized that we live in an awesome place where people take care of each other on all levels. Everybody was involved in raising Spike and me.

After *Getting a Grip* came out, kids began sharing their experiences with us. It seems that everyone does something in their daily diabetes management that can help someone else. This book is a collection of the information we have gleaned from the community of kids with diabetes.

Spike: *Tips for Kids* is a collection of practical tips that *work*. More than 100 kids, along with their parents and doctors, contributed to writing *Tips,* and we bet you can relate to a lot of the experiences that other young people living with diabetes have had. We hope you can use these tips to make your life a little easier and to prepare yourself for new and exciting activities.

P.S. When you find something that really works for you, write it down and share it with other families to help them out. Send your tips to us and, who knows, maybe *you* can be in the next book, helping thousands of kids with diabetes.

Bo and Spike Loy
boandspike@aol.com

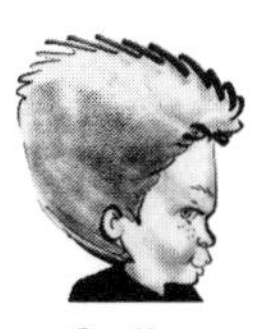

Spike

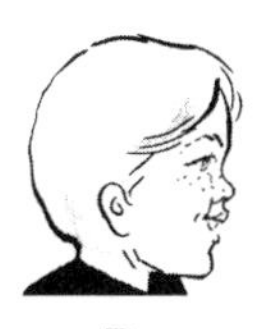

Bo

CHAPTER
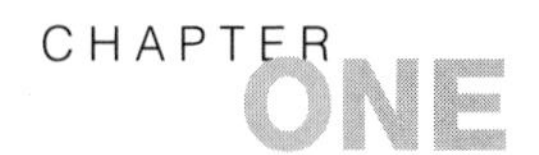

Better Looking and Smarter, Too

Since we wrote *Getting a Grip on Diabetes*, hundreds of kids have shared special tips and techniques with us. Some people deal with their day-to-day diabetes treatment just like we do. Some people have a whole different system that really works well for them. Other kids have had experiences that neither Bo nor I have had in our 32 combined years of diabetes, such as switching to pumps at an early age, going through oral surgery, attending diabetes camp, or being on a college-level sports team. Their stories and ideas are new for us, too.

In *Tips for Kids* we have included tips from kids of all different ages, about all sorts of daily activities and once-in-a-lifetime events. Bo and I use these very same pages for reference whenever something comes up that is new to us. Looking back on it, within these pages is also the story of our journey to going on the pump.

Kids with diabetes are smart kids, geniuses, most of them! Learning about boluses and basals and units (and half-units) and counting carbs, and balancing exercise with insulin and food and Gatorade makes you smart! While we were working on *Tips for Kids*, we met some kids who were helping their parents measure out their insulin dosages when they were 4 years old! We also met teens playing college-level sports (some injecting, some on the pump) who have taken managing their diabetes to a science.

Just read through this book and look at all these amazing tips and techniques for fine-tuning your diabetes, and you'll agree that kids with diabetes are smarter than your average bear. Plus, we're pretty sure diabetes makes us all better looking, too!

Dealing with Low Blood Sugars

When you have low blood sugar, your body alerts you by dumping adrenaline into your bloodstream. The adrenaline causes the shaky, sweaty, and clammy symptoms. The medical term for low blood sugar is *hypoglycemia*. We never say, "I am feeling the symptoms of hypoglycemia," we just say, "I'm low."

What's a low blood sugar feel like? It's a little different for everybody, but we all agree the common signs of a low are:

- Headaches
- Empty stomach
- Feeling dizzy, shaky, sweaty
- Clammy hands
- Crying, getting violently upset, feeling angry
- Inability to make a decision or concentrate on homework
- Speedy talking

Every kid with diabetes has lows. We still get plenty of lows, and we're in our twenties. We are a lot better at preventing them now and a *whole* lot better at treating them so we feel better faster. Whether you are injecting or on the pump, these tips from kids from all over the country will help you deal with lows, too. Some kids use glucose tabs, some use sugary treats, and some, especially pumpers, use "The Rule of 15" (page 222).

- If you feel very low, eat right away—then test.

- If you run out of blood testing strips and you think you are low, don't wait. When in doubt, eat or drink some fast-acting carbs.
- Low blood sugars often occur right before meals, after exercising, when insulin is peaking, and sometimes in the middle of the night.

Tip: I treat low blood sugars with glucose tablets.
–Cory Graham, age 12

Tip: I carry a zip-lock bag in my cooler with Cake Mate Frosting and sugar cubes. If I am really low, 5 sugar cubes work! *–Matt Egizi, age 9*

Tip: To handle lows I eat a little bag of Skittles, the kind you get at Halloween. One bag of Skittles brings me right up, and I really like Skittles. *–Kacie Doyle, age 11*

Tip: Always carry a granola bar. *–Valerie Kintz, age 15*

Tip: I always tell my mom when I don't feel good. Then she tests me, and I eat. *–Karlee Burgess, age 6*
(diagnosed three weeks when she gave this tip.)

Tip: When I feel low, I tell my mom, "I'm hungry."
–Laura Valine, age 5

Tip: When I'm low, I usually say, "I feel funny."
–Derrick Crowe, age 8

Tip: When I feel funny, I eat. *–Karlee Burgess, age 6*

Tip: I like honey packets for my lows. They taste better than that glucose stuff. *–Derrick Crowe, age 8*

Tip: I carry LifeSavers with me in case I get hungry in-between snack times. *–Ben Weber, age 12*

Tip: Always keep a little something to eat with you in case you go low. *–Chris Cisneros, age 14*

Tip: I carry bite-sized Milky Way candy bars. If I feel low, I test. If I'm under 50, I eat one bar, then test 10 minutes later. I also carry glucose tabs in my purse.
–Alexie Milton, age 14

Tip: Try not to eat too much when you are low, it makes you go high afterwards. *–Saira Khan, age 16*

Tip: If you are worried about being low, test.
–Jill Shatkus, age 16

Tip: If your sugar level is high, and you take your shot, you may feel low soon after. When sugar level drops fast, it can make you feel low. A way to avoid feeling low when your sugar is dropping is to eat a few crackers when you inject. *–Saira Khan, age 16*

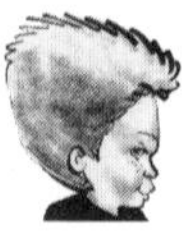

I always eat something after I inject/bolus so I won't experience that sinking feeling when my sugars come down.

Tip: If I'm low in the middle of the night when my mom or dad checks me, my favorite thing is low-fat milk with a tablespoon of sugar-free chocolate and a slice of peanut butter toast. Milk and toast usually bring my blood sugar up to a good number. *–Brittany Brown, age 10*

Tip: If I get low in the middle of the night or while I'm sleeping, it feels like my hands and arms have fallen asleep.
–Mary Costello, age 21

Tip: If you feel low, do something about it!
–Brandon Velilla, age 14

Very low blood sugar can make your body react less to the next low blood sugar. You may not feel the symptoms until your blood sugar drops to an even lower level than the previous low. To fix this, test often and work on having a series of normal blood sugars.

Dealing with High Blood Sugars

Just like lows, high blood sugars are something we all have to deal with. Usually all it takes to bring down a high sugar is a couple of units of fast-acting insulin or a quick bolus from your pump. When we were kids, if one of us was high, my mom would give whoever was high a shot, give us both water, and tell us both to go run around the house 10 times. Seems crazy, but it worked. When you have more sugar in your blood than normal, doctors call it *hyperglycemia*. We just say, "I'm high."

What's a high blood sugar feel like? It can be different for everyone. Some common signs of high blood sugar are:

- Headaches
- Thirst
- Energy loss
- Feeling hyper
- Speedy talking
- Peeing frequently
- Having clear pee

No matter how good your control is, sometimes you will just have some high blood sugars. It could be because you took less insulin than you needed for a meal, your insulin is old, you are sick, or because of hormones in your body that you have no way of controlling. Highs happen.

- Check your blood sugar. If you are high, adjust your blood sugar by taking a small amount of rapid-acting insulin. A good rule of thumb is that one unit of insulin (H, N, or R) can take care of about 40 points of blood sugar. (Everyone's body reacts a little differently.)
- If you inject insulin to help come down, be sure to check your sugar again an hour or two later. If you haven't come down, you might need a little bit more. If you are coming down fast, you should have a quick snack, like half a sandwich, so you don't end up low!
- Once you get the hang of it, don't be afraid to adjust your dose on your own a little bit to deal with highs.

Tip: If you are high, 15 to 30 minutes of exercise can really help you start to come down. *–Jessica Lopez, age 16*

Tip: Drink lots of water when your sugar is high.
–Katherine Gresch, age 16

Tip: Drinking lots of water will help keep you hydrated and is an easy way to help yourself feel better.
–A.J. Fenner, age 18

Tip: When I am running high, like on the weekends, I drink a lot of water and eat a little less.
–Herbert Larkin, age 17

Tip: It is better to be a little bit high rather than low.
–Rory Tarbox, age 19

Tip: If you have lots of highs in a row (like almost every test for three or four days), call your doc and talk about adjusting your insulin dosage. *–Kenna Connell, age 16*

Tip: If I get dizzy . . . have a headache, or feel nauseated, I suspect high blood sugar. Then I test at my desk. If I'm 190 or higher, I take some fast-acting insulin—0.8 units. If I'm between 200 and 250, I take 1 unit. One unit of fast-acting insulin brings my blood sugar down 50 points. It is different for everyone. You learn by trial and error. *–Nick Brown, age 13*

Tip: If your sugars are running high because you're sick or because of hormones and you increase your dosage to come back down, watch out for lows! Once your body gets back to normal, your new, increased dosage may be too much. *That's how Spike and I know when we aren't really sick anymore—our sugars come back down! –Bo*

Tip: Change insulin bottles. A lot of times when I am running high consistently, it is because my insulin has lost its potency. When I suspect this to be the case, I just throw out my old bottles and open new ones. Be aware that new insulin has a kick. *–Nick Brown, age 13*

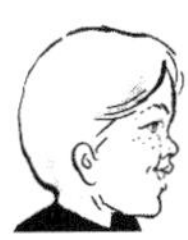

New insulin has a kick! That's the perfect way to say it!

Tip: My mom throws opened insulin out after 4 weeks. *–Sarah Dorsey, age 3*

Watch for ketones!

When you are running high or feeling lousy, check for ketones, especially when you are on the pump (page 132).

Testing routine

Jessica: Testing is part of my routine. I probably test 10 times a day. I have regular test times, like before I eat and before bed, but I also test whenever I feel high. When I'm high, I can't think properly. I know I'm high when I feel groggy and gross, or I get a weird taste in my mouth that doesn't go away even when I brush my teeth. I can be going along feeling totally normal, and within minutes, I can feel totally tired. That's an indication that I'm high, so I test.

I drink water when I'm high and often go on a walk. If I'm over 300, I take a little fast-acting insulin and just lie down and relax for a few minutes until my numbers come down. It usually takes 15 to 30 minutes. Sometimes, if I'm really high and not feeling well, I disconnect my pump and use a syringe to take a shot of fast-acting insulin. It seems to work faster for me.

–Jessica Stogsdill, age 18

Tip: Your heart beats faster when you have high blood sugar (hyperglycemia). And I have noticed that when you have super high blood sugar, the drop of blood from a finger prick appears thick and dark. With super low blood sugar (hypoglycemia), the drop of blood often appears light colored and runny. *–Jessica Stogsdill, age 18*

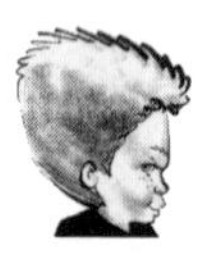

We noticed that too. Thought we were the only ones. . . .

Tip: When you are having a series of high sugars and having trouble figuring out why, it is a sign that it is time to see your doctor. *–Thomas Lee, age 11*

Organizing Things

Being organized is the key to handling diabetes. If you keep all of your food and supplies in the same place every day and follow a routine, diabetes just becomes a small, easy-to-manage part of your life.

- Be organized at home.
- Have a routine that's easy to follow.
- Keep your diabetes supplies in a drawer in the kitchen (the *Diabetes Drawer*).
- Keep extra *back-up* supplies around.
- Keep your insulin in the butter shelf in the fridge (the *Insulin Shelf*).
- Put your kit on the same shelf in the fridge each time you walk in the door.
- Keep low-fat milk in the fridge. It's good for treating low blood sugar.
- Have a shelf in the pantry stocked with your special snack foods (the *Low Food Shelf*). Keep sick day foods there, too (real 7-Up and Gatorade).
- Take your kit and cooler whenever you go out.

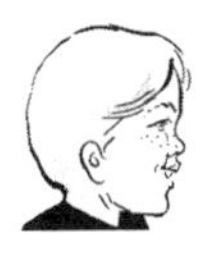

All our friends know the low food shelf is off-limits to them and is there in case we need it!

Away from home

Tip: B-I-F-T: Bracelet, Insulin, Food, Tester.

–Jenna Rohm, age 16

Tip: Put a granola bar in your pocket when you leave the house.

–Evan McMillin, age 10

Tip: Always carry a few dollars so you can buy food if you need it.

–Chris Cisneros, age 14

Tip: I always carry glucose tabs in my backpack.

–Mo Lopez, age 10

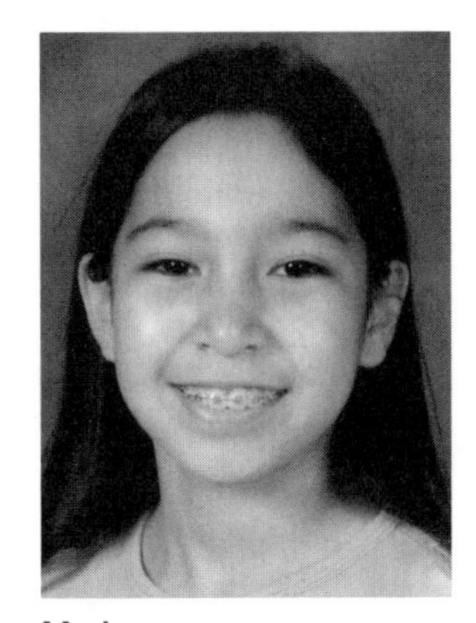

Mo Lopez

Tip: Put candy in your purse. *–Katie Tucker, age 13*

Tip: Carry juice on you when you are away from home. *–Stephen Whitlock, age 16*

Tip: Always take your back-up food into stores and malls. It is a hassle to have to go back to the car when you need a snack. *–Andrew Rieger, age 12*

Tip: Take your glucagon kit on overnight trips. Whenever I spend the night at my grandma's, I ask her, "Do you have food in the fridge?" *–Christian Cooper, age 10*

Tip: Keep a copy of glucagon instructions in your kit or cooler (page 253). *–Bo*

Tip: When going to a remote area, like on a bike ride away from home, take a buddy to look after you in case of an emergency! *–Brian Feinzimer, age 13*

Tip: When you go somewhere alone, wear a diabetes notification necklace or bracelet. *–Alex Edwards, age 14*

Tip: My mom and dad carry all our back-up supplies in the insulated bag we got at PADRE. It goes everywhere I go. *–Mo Lopez, age 10*

Tip: I keep my supplies in my backpack. *–Cameron Olson, age 5*

Tip: Whenever I travel anywhere, I bring back-up insulin and needles. *–Herbert Larkin, age 17*

Tip: Make sure your nanny/caregiver has a snack in their car. *–Sophie Sheridan, age 9*

Tip: Take more supplies than you think you will need. *–Stacy Gemmell, age 19*

Tip: If you spend a lot of time at a relative's home, keep a full set of supplies there including a cooler full of snacks. *–Benjamin Siegel, age 7*

Tip: I always carry a cell phone. It makes things so much easier. *–Valerie Kintz, age 15*

Tailgate picnics

On our family outings, we pack a picnic. We all eat the same foods together out of the trunk of our car. That way we never have to wait in lines for food and always have the opportunity to talk. We love our tailgate parties.

–Andrew Rieger, age 12

Food: One of our favorite things

Eating (and sometimes not eating) is a big part of taking care of yourself and your diabetes. The most important thing we can tell you about food is this: Make sure you always have some around. Always. Immediate access to food will help make life go smoothly. It takes a while to get into the habit of always having food around, so we talk about food a lot.

- Always carry food
  - In your pocket
  - In your cooler/backpack
  - In your car
  - In any car you are riding in
  - In your mom's purse and your dad's briefcase

When you're injecting insulin, you match your carbohydrates to the insulin in your system so you don't crash. Because it

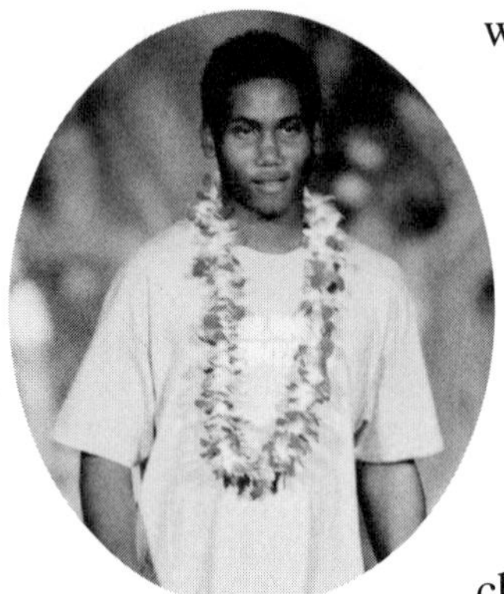
Herbert Larkin

worked for us, we always ate protein with our carbs. When we were little, we divided food into categories that we called short, medium, and long. Short-lasting foods are fruit juice, milk, and sugary things. Medium-lasting foods are bread, crackers, pasta, and cereal. Long-lasting foods are string cheese, jerky, meat, chicken, eggs, and nuts.

On the pump the constant short-acting insulin entering your system, the basal rate, can be set so low that you do not have to constantly keep food in your system. Then each time you eat, you dial in bursts of short-acting insulin to cover the carbs. You have to learn how to count carbs, but it's pretty easy (pages 234–235).

On injections we were constantly chasing lows and treating highs. In talking to our friends, we learned that you spend less time chasing lows with food when you are on the pump.

Snacks

Keep a supply of snack food around the house so you can grab some whenever you leave the house. Blood sugars bounce around more when you are young and growing, which means you need to check your sugars (glucose level) and snack more often.

Snacks when you need sugar (carbohydrates)

Tip: I like Hansen's Junior Juice, apple juice, mixed fruit, and fruit punch. (This snack juice has exactly 15 grams of carb.) *–Eric Koch, age 3*

Tip: I like to eat Halloween-sized candy bars when I am low. (Each bar has 10–20 grams of carbs. Check the package.) *–Hayley Kucia, age 6*

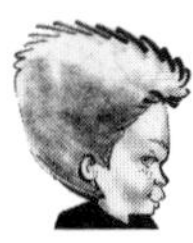

What a great way to put all the Halloween candy to use.

Tip: I like it when my mom gets a fruit drink and pours it in miniature ice cube trays and freezes them. I like to eat them on a hot day. *–Andrew Simecka, age 8*

Tip: Our favorite snacks are crackers and fruit rollups. *–Chris and Cory Graham, ages 11 and 12*

Tip: I always carry a mini juice. *–Mo Lopez, age 10*
(Libby's Juicy Juice, 4 oz, 15 carbs; Hansen's Jr. Juice, 4 oz, 15 carbs)

Tip: The sugar tablets at SaveOn Drugs taste good. They taste like Giant Smarties. *–Colin Prothero, age 18*

Tip: Mix bottled Gatorade with water when you exercise. This will keep you from getting low and help keep you from getting high. Plus you only have to buy half as much Gatorade! *–Andy Savage, age 15*

Tip: My favorite snacks are green apples, cheese, and peanut butter and juice. *–Hayley Kucia, age 6*

Tip: My favorite snack is pretzels. *–Wiley Newman, Jr. aka Grey Wolf, age 8 1/2*
(His dad says he likes them too—low carb, no sugar, and low fat.)

Tip: I like to snack on chips, granola bars and Power Bars. *–Alexie Milton, age 14*

Tip: Some good carbohydrate snacks are: orange slices, Charleston Chews, apple juice, and Capri Sun.

–Cory Graham, age 12

Tip: We like little bags of Goldfish crackers.

–Steven Guzman and Abel Guzman, ages 7 and 9

Tip: I like pizza—no sauce. *–Carson Canada, age 5*

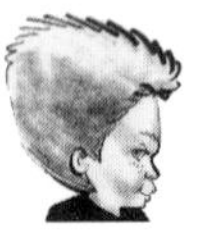

I hated sauce too, until I was 19. Never even realized I was cutting some of the carbs out of pizza!

Tip: At snack time, I have a Baby Ruth granola bar [28 grams of carb] or a Kudo granola bar [16–18 grams of carb] and a piece of fruit, depending on how many carbs I need. *–Evan McMillin, age 10*

Tip: Dreyers makes the best ice cream—no sugar added.

–Wiley Newman, Jr. aka Grey Wolf, age 8

Kid Recipe—Ice Cream Substitute

This is my delicious ice cream substitute. It tastes great, has fewer carbs than ice cream, and is easy to make! Simply mix:

- 1 Tbsp peanut butter
- 1 cup fat-free chocolate pudding (ready-made in little cups)
- 1 cup fat-free Cool Whip

You can put it in a cone, refrigerate, or freeze this treat.

–Stephanie Speer

Snacks when you don't need sugar

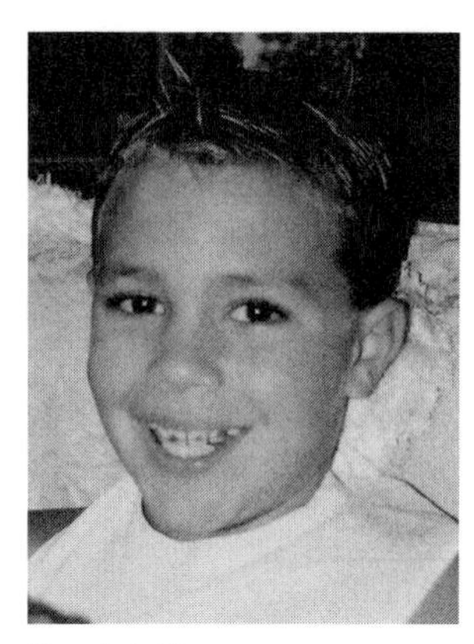
Derrick Crowe

Tip: Propel tastes real good—orange is the best kind

–Derrick Crowe, 8

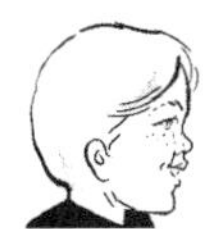

We heard about Propel for the first time from Derrick. It's Gatorade's new flavored water—just 3 carbs per 8 oz!

Tip: I like Crystal Light (zero carbs). *–Jordan White, age 4*

Tip: When you just have to eat something sweet, but don't need it (you're not low, you're just craving sugar) a tablespoon of Cool Whip works pretty well. Have your mom freeze some in ice trays, then pop one out every once in a while. It has a good carb count (1 carb per tablespoon). *–Natalie Bayne, age 10*

I Scream, You Scream, We All Scream for . . . Cool Whip?

When I was little, my parents would give me Cool Whip when I wanted ice cream, and I didn't know that it *wasn't* ice cream. They put Cool Whip in a cake cone, so it was practically a free food—hardly any carbs. And it was a treat for me!

–Brittany Rausch, age 15

➠ **Note:** The regular sized cake cone has 3 carbs compared to a sugar cone with 10 carbs!

Tip: I like to snack on string cheese, beef jerky, and sugar-free Jello. *–Samantha McGuigan, age 8*

Lunch for the little folks

When we were in grade school on injections at every snack and meal, we ate carbohydrates combined with protein. Combining carbohydrates and protein helped us avoid big blood sugar spikes. Some of our favorite lunches were:

- String cheese, jerky, banana, and milk
- A burrito with scrambled eggs, sausage, and milk
- Cold fried chicken, crackers, string cheese, nuts, and milk

Tip: I like to eat turkey bologna with a piece of Iron Kids Crustless Bread. (2 slices, 17 grams of carb)

–Eric Koch, age 3

Tip: I like peanut butter and jelly sandwiches.

–Sara Morda, age 4

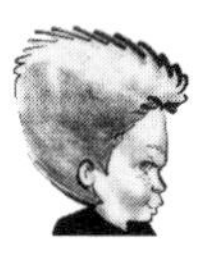

So do we!

Tip: I like to eat little hot dogs on toothpicks, or roast beef, pickles, and a little piece of garlic bread.

–Laura Valine, age 5

Tip: I like to eat something different for lunch every day, like a tuna sandwich or a hot dog. *–Hayley Kucia, age 6*

Tip: I like macaroni and cheese with tuna and peas and a glass of whole milk for lunch. It makes my numbers fantastic. *–Christian Cooper, age 10*

Tip: I love vegetables and often eat vegetables, fruit, smoked ham or turkey, and a diet drink for lunch.

–Stacie Hardin, age 13

Bedtime snacks

Our friend, Dr. Ronald Chochinov, recommends Extend Bars (converts to glucose over nine hours) and Glucerna Bars (converts to glucose over 4 hours) to help kids avoid middle-of-the-night lows. These bars are made with cornstarch, so they dissolve into your system slowly. If you are having nighttime lows, try eating a bar at bedtime.

Tip: Always eat something before going to bed. Toast with peanut butter, string cheese, or cereal and milk are some good ideas. *–Kenna Connell, age 16*

Tip: Before bed I eat green apples and peanut butter or crackers and peanut butter or cottage cheese and fruit.

–Hayley Kucia, age 6

Tip: Before bed I like apples and peanut butter, and watermelon and string cheese. *–Marissa Williams, age 4*

Kelly's Bedtime Snack

My favorite bedtime snack is ice cream. I'm so active I can handle the carbs. I also like to put light vanilla yogurt on top of graham crackers for a bedtime snack or have Goldfish crackers with a glass of milk.

–Kelly Hrubeniuk, age 10

Tip: My favorite bedtime snacks are Danimals and applesauce sticks. *–Jordan White, age 4*
(Dannon drinkable lowfat yogurt, 3.1 oz bottles, 16 carbs. Squeeze N Go Applesauce sticks, 14 grams carb.)

Eric Koch, age 3, is on the pump so he doesn't always need a nighttime snack. But when he does, he likes Yoplait Gogurt, 13 grams of carb in one tube. Gogurt has 2 grams of fat and 2 grams of protein, too.

Eating out at restaurants

Spike: Eating out at a restaurant can be a little tricky, because you never know when your food will be served. Sometimes they might even lose your order. When I go out to eat on a date (or when I am too lazy to cook), I follow the same routine every time. I test right after I am seated.

If I'm low, I eat a granola bar—either the one that is always in my pocket or the one that I keep in my insulin kit. When the waiter comes to take the drink order, I request bread or crackers or chips right away. Sometimes I order regular soda or orange juice. If I'm really low, I go out to my car and raid my cooler—then I go back inside. A couple of times when we were kids and I was low, my mom tracked down the waiter and told him I had diabetes and had to eat right away. I got dessert before dinner.

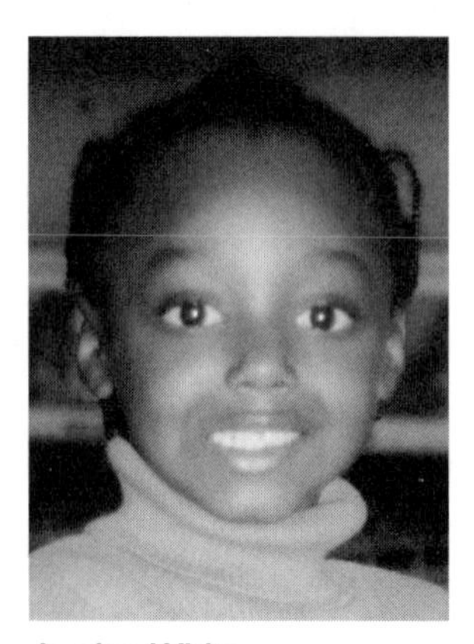
Jordan White

If I'm high, I order a more protein-y meal. I skip the potato or fries. I don't, however, take insulin until my food arrives. If you take a whole bunch of insulin and come down, and it takes an hour to get your food, you can crash. *Only if I am really high and there is already bread on the table do I ever take any insulin at*

One Simple Rule for Eating Out

Never take any insulin before your food is served *unless* your blood sugar is very high and you have something to eat (like bread or chips) already on the table.

all before my food is served. This goes for pumpers, too. Don't bolus before your food arrives.

Tip: Always carry a granola bar in your pocket, even at restaurants where you are going to order food anyway.
–Spike

Tip: Wait until your food is served, then inject your insulin or bolus. If I'm low, I take my insulin after my food arrives. If I'm high, I take it when I get the appetizer.
–Steven Whitlock, age 16

Tip: If you get low while waiting for food in a restaurant, go ahead and tell an employee you need sugar, like a *real* Coke, right now! *–Stacy Gemmell, age 19*

Spike: Always keep a granola bar in your kit. It's a good backup for when the one in your pocket is a little too melty and smashed up. (Then remember to put a new one in your kit and grab a new, un-smashed one for your pocket. Give the melty, smashed one to a friend—it's the thought that counts!)

Bo: Plan your fast food according to your activity level. If you're going surfing, go ahead and have a bean burrito at Taco Bell. If you're going back to school to sit at a desk, have the beef taco and a diet drink.

Junk Food

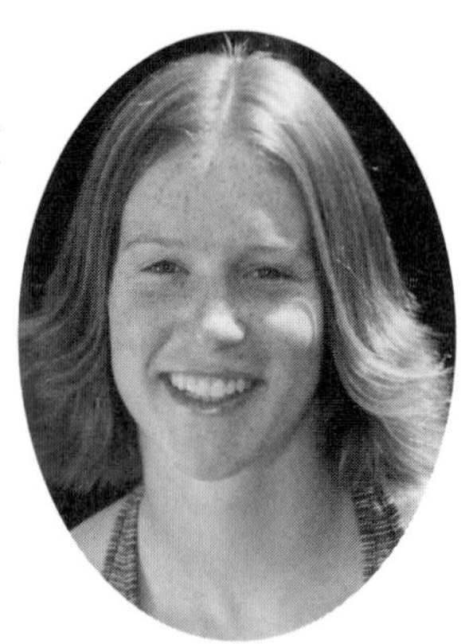
Blair Ryan

I eat junk food, within reason. I rarely eat at fast-food places, not because I have diabetes, but because it is not all that appealing to me. I am, though, a sucker for ice cream. I treat ice cream just like any other food.

The pump makes eating anything easy. I just think, "Okay how many grams of carbohydrate does it have? How much insulin do I need to cover it?" I cover all junk food with my insulin-to-carb ratio. I take 1 unit of insulin to 1 carb exchange (carb exchanges are servings of food that contain 15 grams of carbohydrate). Everyone's insulin-to-carb ratio is different. Because I run so much (page 223), I have pretty high insulin sensitivity. I treat junk food just like any other food—count the carbs and cover with insulin.

–Blair Ryan, age 16

Spike: If you don't need the extra carbs, when you order a hamburger, hold the sauce, skip the fries, and drink diet soda.

Tell Everyone You Know That You Have Diabetes!

Bo: I met Brittany at a PADRE meeting in Orange County, California. She is an awesome, outgoing, modest girl, who is very involved in helping other kids. Brittany is an original member of a singing group, *The Pump Girls*. Every member of the group has diabetes and is on the pump. They perform all over, plus they have produced a CD. Brittany sent her tips in this e-mail:

> Hi Bo, this is Brittany. I see myself as a girl who just happens to have had diabetes since she was two. I have always been open about it. Each year in elementary school I would present my diabetes to my new class at show-and-tell. I would explain a little about diabetes, do my blood sugar, and then draw up a shot and explain that.
>
> When you are a kid, telling other kids about diabetes helps you connect with them. Kids would ask questions and sometimes I would even bring extra lancets and let the kids do their own blood sugars. When the kids interacted, they felt like they knew me better, understood what I was going through, and became a part of my life.
>
> Try to be open about your diabetes, because most people are interested and want to know about it. Just about everybody has an aunt or friend or someone they know who has D.
>
> *–Brittany Rausch, age 15*

Make your parents part of your team

When you need help—ask. Some parents want to do it all, while others want their kids to do everything. If you are doing everything and you get exhausted—or just tired and frustrated—talk to your mom or dad. Ask them to give you a little mental break. Set a time limit. Let them do the thinking for a while. A little break may be just what the doctor ordered to help get you back on track and ready to take control again.

Tip: If your parents or grandparents have trouble reading the markings on your syringes you can help them out. Get a syringe magnifier (MagniGuide) at the pharmacy.

–Samantha McGuigan, age 8

It's a Team Effort

Here's a great story about letting everyone around you know about your diabetes, so they can help. This is an example of the right way to do it.

Julia: The minute I was diagnosed I called my rowing teammates from the hospital. They were incredibly supportive from day one, visiting me at the hospital, learning about blood sugar, and glucagon. When I returned to practice, my teammates looked out for me. My parents told my coach I had diabetes, and he agreed to carry extra supplies and be aware of my symptoms in case of lows or highs.

My parents accompanied me for the first week back at practice, so they could help me front-load (calorie up) and talk to the coaches. Our rowing community was very close, so everyone knew I had diabetes. My coxswains were especially helpful. (The coxswain sits at the helm and directs the rowers. [Don't worry, I didn't know what a coxswain was either. –Spike]) They carried my juice in the boat and were always alert to see if I needed anything. At times it feels like a bit of a chore to explain everything about diabetes, but I always relaxed when I knew that I was surrounded by caring people.

–Julia Halprin Jackson, age 18

- Always alert your coach, teammates, friends, classmates, and teachers that you have diabetes. Tell them about your symptoms and emergency information.
- Give your coach a copy of Symptoms (page 250).

CHAPTER TWO

Exercise and Sports

Everyone's Favorite Thing to Do!

We exercise every day to feel well and to maintain level sugars. Try to look at your body like a machine. Think about how much fuel (carbohydrates) it needs to complete a task. Then do something you like to do. Kevon Hannam is a skateboarder. He loves it, and skates every day. Kevon's advice is: Have fun and take care of yourself!

Tip: Carry a little money when you are skating, so you can buy stuff when you need it. Carry water and Gatorade in your backpack. *–Kevon Hannam, age 13*

Tip: Don't be afraid to go out and play sports. Be a regular kid. You'll soon figure out how to balance your insulin intake. *–Nick Brown, age 13*

Tip: Play sports—just always make sure you have sugar and extra food with you at all times. If you feel low during a game, come to the sidelines, eat a snack, and go on with the game. *–Laura Reichstadt, age 14*

It's Such a Simple Idea

Mary: It's such a simple idea. I used to think that exercise simply meant you had to eat more. Then I realized that the more insulin you have circulating in your bloodstream, the more chance you have of getting low. *Exercise enhances the delivery of insulin.* It makes it work quicker and more efficiently. I have learned to reduce my insulin before I exercise. I can lower my pump's basal rate a couple of hours before practice or a meet. This way I am taking almost no insulin at all before and during heavy exercise.

–Mary Costello, age 21

When you exercise, your muscles warm up. Warm muscles absorb more sugar. This means: When you are exercising, you will require less insulin or more carbs.

Tip: In the beginning, test before, during, and after sports. Once you get the hang of it, you'll be able to adjust your insulin down a bit while snacking during play.
–Hannah Smith, age 11

Tip: It's good to build muscle mass. Muscles absorb sugar and help keep blood sugars level even when you aren't actually doing the exercise. *–Brandon Velilla, age 14*

Tip: I eat extra before a sports event. *–Chris Cisneros, age 14*

Tip: Do a glucose test before you exercise to make sure you're not low. If it's normal, eat a small snack, so your sugar doesn't go low later. *–Saira Khan, age 16*

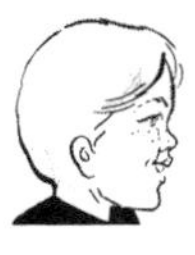

That's a great tip. If your blood sugar is right where you like it to be during rest times, it is too low for exercising. A quick snack is what you need before getting in the game.

Tip: While you are exercising, take a water bottle of diluted Gatorade and drink it regularly. *–Andy Savage, age 15*

Tip: If you get overheated, your sugars can drop to low levels fast. *–Sam Rodriguez, age 15*

Tip: No matter what sport or exercise you do, always make sure you eat a good meal before exercising and always have something on you in case you get low blood sugar. When I go for walks (2–2 1/2 miles) I carry LifeSavers, juice, and, depending on how far I go, my cell phone.

–Jennifer Ogden, age 19

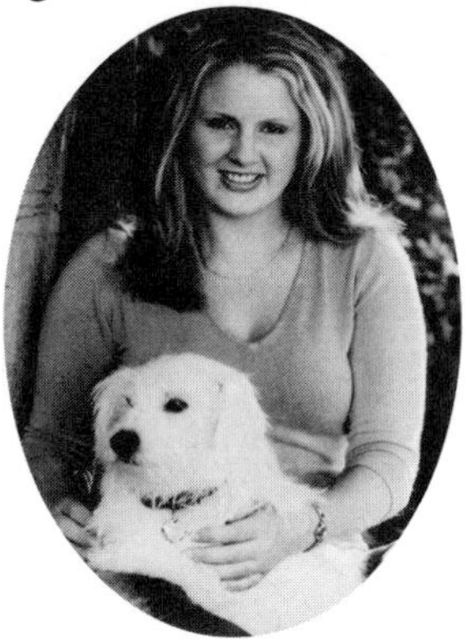

Jennifer Ogden

Hot water tips

Tip: Because the insulin absorption rate soars in hot water, don't inject insulin or bolus right before you get into a hot tub or hot bath. *–Clare Rosenfeld, age 16*

Tip: Detach your pump when you are going to sit in a hot tub. Insulin is very sensitive to heat. Hot water will ruin it. *–Clare Rosenfeld, age 16*

Tip: Watch those long hot showers after exercising. It can be harder to sense a low in a hot bath, hot shower, or soaking in a hot tub. The same goes if you are sitting down watching a really intense movie—adrenaline can lower your blood sugar, and you won't know it.

–Clare Rosenfeld, age 16

Tip: Don't hop into a hot bath when you are low. Hot water can speed up the action of insulin. *–James Neil, age 12*

Water Sports and the Pump

Emily Stahlman, 10, is in the water a lot, sometimes for 4–5 hours at a time. She has learned to disconnect her pump and cap the infusion site before swim practice or a meet. Sometimes she takes a quick bolus before she disconnects. Emily checks her sugar every hour or so while she swims, reconnects for a quick spurt (when needed), and she is off again.

Emily: The pump has been good for me, especially with my active life. One nice thing about the pump: when you are exercising, your lows don't tend to be as low. The pump has really helped cut down on the number of lows I have when I am swimming competitively. In fact, I just qualified for the State Swim Championships!

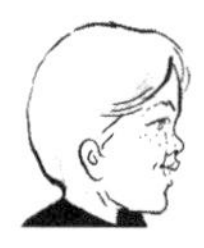

Wow, Spike's proud of his swimming ability . . . and he only doggie paddles!

Another handy thing I use to keep the infusion set in place when I am in and out of the water frequently, like day-long swim competitions, is very sticky Mastisol on my skin, under the infusion site tape.

- You can give yourself your basal rate just before disconnecting. If you are very active, you may not need it.
- When you go swimming, disconnect your pump, and put a cap on the infusion site.

- When you take your pump off at the pool, lake, or beach, put it in a cooler in the shade, away from the sand.
- Swimming is one exercise that can cause delayed low blood sugar. Sometimes I run a lower temporary basal rate for 12–24 hours after a day of competition.

–Emily Stahlman, age 10

Tip: I love to wear my pump in a pump pouch around my waist. It is comfortable, and I can run around and play and not worry about my pump. My mom makes them in many colors and prints, so I always have a fun selection to choose from (www.pump-pouch.com). This is how I make pumping fun! *–Tessa Davidson, age 6*

Tip: You can personalize your pump. I decorate mine with stickers. *–Sophie Sheridan, age 9*

Tip: **Pumps don't float!** Don't wake-board or water-ski with a pump . . . even if it's waterproof! It will fly off and sink and cost $5,000 to replace! (There is a nice pump on the bottom of Lake Powell!) *–George Munson, age 11*

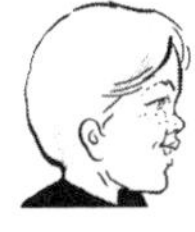

Now that's a funny tip!

Individual Sports

Surfing

Bo: Embrace a sport, make it yours. Exercise builds muscle mass and burns calories and works to keep your sugars down. Sports do more than just make you physically healthy, they make you feel good. My favorite sport is surfing!

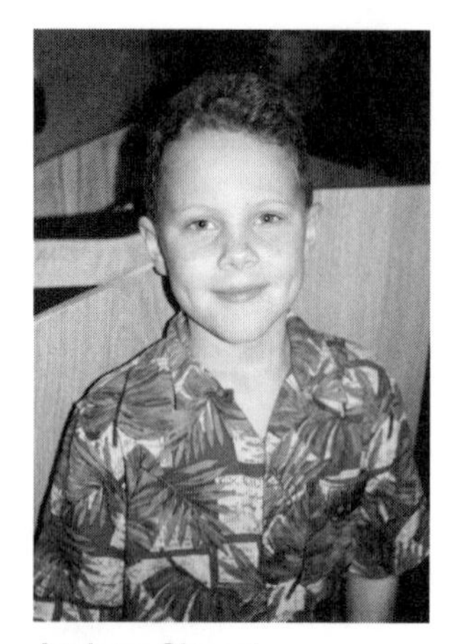
Andrew Simecka

From the minute I dropped into my first wave, surfing has been an important part of my life. During the school year, after a week of tests and quizzes, projects and essays, deadlines and obligations, I can feel a little overwhelmed. Surfing really clears my head and helps me to relax. There's nothing like paddling through the cool ocean waters on a hot sunny day, gliding across a glassy face, or dipping my hand into a glistening wave. Once I'm up, nothing else matters, all my worries are left behind. Spike feels the same way.

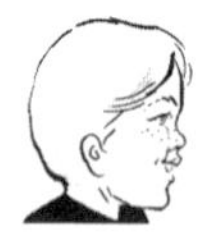

Diabetes ever get you down? Find a sport or hobby that you love and just forget about whatever's bugging you for a while.

- Water sports require more vigilance.
- Never surf alone.
- Eat before you go out.
- Put a tube of Cake Mate frosting or glucose gel in your trunks pocket. Wearing a wetsuit? Put it in your sleeve.
- Come in every hour for to eat and do a blood test.
- If you get low when you are out in the lineup, ask someone to paddle in with you.
- Always have a cooler with food waiting for you on the beach. Keep it closed so dogs and birds (or the occasional cow) don't get into your food.
- Cold water and exhaustion lower blood sugars rapidly. Have plenty of carbs in your cooler on the shore.

Tip: I lower my short-acting insulin by 1/4 before I go surfing. *–Ant Engeln, age 14*

Tip: I take a little soft cooler down to the beach with ice pack, juice, and granola bars, and I put my pump in there to keep it cool and out of the sand. Also, take money so you can buy food after a day of surfing.

–Andy Savage, age 15

Dirt bike riding

Jessica: When I ride dirt bikes, I put my pump in the front of my sports bra because I probably won't fall flat on my face. It happens once in a while but not often. When I get ready to ride, I always stick some glucose tablets and a Power Bar in my pocket or boots. When riding with my family, I feel secure that they can help fast if I need it, but if we are out in the middle of nowhere or riding in the desert, I always carry food.

I have the ice chest Spike and Bo gave me years ago, and I take it on all bike trips filled with juice, beef jerky, peanuts (I love peanuts), and Power Bars. Tiger Milk Bars work well, too. I leave my cooler at the campground or wherever we are staying. Just before we head out, I check my blood sugar for sure. If we're riding in desert, I carry a fanny pack with my meter, Power Bars, and glucose tabs. My mom always carries glucose tablets, Power Bars, and juice.

Our favorite place to ride is in the sand at Pismo Beach, California. We put paddle tires on the back to keep the bikes from being squirrelly and flipping out. Without the paddles, you're just constantly digging a hole in the sand.

Motorcycle riding, especially riding in the sand, requires a lot of bodywork. It's not like you are just sitting there and giving it gas—you burn a lot of calories—so I make a point of riding back to camp every 45 minutes to test and eat something, especially if it's hot. *When it's hot outside, you go low faster,* so I have a snack every 45 minutes, like clockwork.

- When you're riding dirt bikes, stick some glucose tablets and a Power Bar in your boot.
- Consider the distance you'll be traveling and carry enough food with you, so you can walk back to camp if your bike breaks down.
- Carry your kit in your saddle pack.
- Carry Gatorade and snacks.
- If you are going for a long ride, let your friends carry some of your back-up food.
- Keep a packed cooler at your base camp.
- Tell your riding friends about your diabetes. Give them a copy of *Symptoms,* so if you go low, they can help (page 250).
- Tape a copy of *Symptoms* in the top of your cooler. That way if there's an accident or if you get low, your friends will know how to help.
- Take glucagon on dirt bike-riding trips. Keep it in the RV or at base camp. *Jessica Stogsdill, age 18*

Snorkeling

Jennifer: When I am intent on snorkeling I can lose track of time and get low, so I always have some sugar with me out in the ocean. I like to put LifeSavers in my wetsuit sleeve. They get wet, but they stay in place. Some people carry frosting. If you know you're going to be doing a lot of physical activity, you can lower your insulin dose. I keep my insulin kit in the shade on shore.

- Eat a big lunch before snorkeling.
- Tell the people with you that you have diabetes.
- Carry LifeSavers (or frosting) in the sleeve of your wetsuit.
- Keep a snack on the beach in your cooler or backpack.

–Jennifer Ogden, age 19

Weight lifting tips

Spike: I met Brandon Velilla at a PADRE Foundation teen retreat at UCLA. He kept trying to get me to go work out with him during our free activity time, and I promised him I would. I never made it to the gym, though. The problem is that even though he's eight years younger, I'm pretty sure Brandon can bench more weight than I can. I told him I had to go supervise at the pool instead. . . . Anyway, I asked Brandon for a tip on weightlifting, and he e-mailed back:

> Hey Spike,
> It's Brandon. You asked me about your blood sugar dropping hours after doing a hard workout. If you do a very hard workout and don't want your blood sugar to drop right after you finish, either drink a protein shake (such as whey protein powder mixed with milk or water) or eat a protein bar. This should level out your blood sugar for a few hours. I hope this helps you out.
>
> *–Brandon Velilla, age 14*

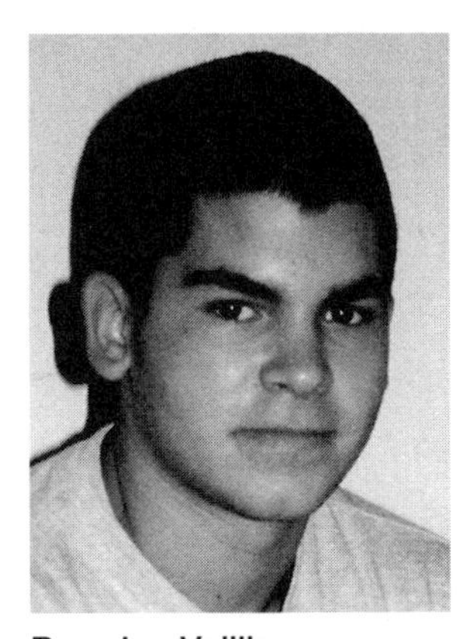

Brandon Velilla

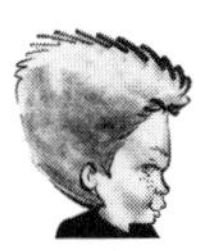

Building muscle mass is great for diabetes. Muscles burn through carbs, so putting on more muscle will help keep your sugars down and level.

Team Sports

Lacrosse

Brooks: Growing up, I loved sports and never let diabetes keep me from playing. In high school I played three sports, and now I play lacrosse at Stanford. Playing on a sports team, especially one that travels, just means that you have to plan ahead. At practice and games, on buses and airplanes, I bring my kit. I make sure that I have plenty of test strips and glucose tablets, and that I have both back-up insulin vials and a glucagon syringe. All of these things are essential, because intense exercise can send mixed signals about hyperglycemia and hypoglycemia (highs and lows).

- If you ever feel strange, TEST!

  Make sure that your coach, trainer, and other players on the team know about your diabetes and what they should do in case you have a reaction. Make sure that the trainer, especially, knows about the glucagon syringe and how to use it. If you've taken all of the precautions, then you should have no trouble.
- Tell your coach you have diabetes.
- Take your glucagon kit to games.

–Brooks Kincaid, age 21

Spike: I met Brooks during fraternity rush, and saw him pull out his One Touch Ultra to check his blood sugar before raiding the free hot wings. With an attitude like his, it's no wonder he is able to do so much and still pass his classes at Stanford.

Rory: Playing lacrosse is a demanding activity that takes a lot of attention. Throughout high school and now in college, I have had to be careful with both what I eat and how much insulin to take. Always follow these two rules: Make sure your blood sugar is regulated while playing any sport and check your blood consistently. This is the regimen I usually follow:

- I check several hours before I play and eat some good food that can carry me through the day. I also usually go easy on the amount of insulin I take because I know that once I start playing, and even for a while after, the need for insulin will be much lower.
- I check about an hour before the actual game to make sure I am not dropping. If I am, I drink some sort of high-sugar drink, like Gatorade or orange juice.
- I check my blood sugar again right before game time. I like to make sure I'm a little bit higher than normal because my blood sugar will begin to drop shortly after beginning play.
- I always drink juice or Gatorade, even after the game is over, because you may continue to drop. Don't worry about high blood sugars (180–240 mg/dl) during sports, because it is safer to be a little high than to be low and risk passing out during a game.

–Rory Tarbox, age 19, plays for USC

Softball

Hannah: I love competitive sports, and I don't let diabetes stop me from doing what I love. I'm 11 years old and have had diabetes for three and a half years. I am also on the pump. This year in softball, I played on Little League Majors and All-Stars teams, and an ASA (Amateur Softball Association) tournament team. So I have had many chances to find out what works for me during games and tournaments.

My first rule is *testing, testing, and testing—before, during, and after*. I keep my pump on during games. During game breaks and while I sit out, I usually have a Jolly Rancher or some kind of little candy.

Once while I was up to bat, the umpire asked me what my pump was. I told him, but I got rattled and struck out. That's why before the game it's a good idea that either you or your coach let the ump know that you have diabetes and you wear a pump. Even if you forget to let him know and he asks what it is, don't get rattled—just tell him, and play your game.

–Hannah Smith, age 11

Tip: Since getting diabetes, I have thrown a perfect game and a no-hitter! Play sports!

–Danny Weiss, age 14

Basketball tips

Hannah: Playing basketball I had a whole different routine than the one for softball, except *for testing, testing, and testing—before, during, and after.* Since basketball is so much more active than softball, it is especially important to test during the games. Also I didn't keep my pump on because of so much more activity.

After basketball games, I tended to go low more often, so my mom and I lowered my after-game basal. It seemed to work real well. Everyone is different, but my plan worked for me. I know, because in 35 basketball games and 60 softball games, I went low only once.

–Hannah Smith, age 11

Valerie: I keep a special bag in my gym bag filled with Gatorade, crackers, and glucose gel. Because basketball is a contact sport, I try to put my pump set where it won't get hot. I usually put it on my leg (on the side of my thigh, along the seam line, and just below the bikini line). While I'm playing basketball, I detach my pump and leave it wrapped up in my jeans inside my athletic bag under the players' bench.

Before the game, I go up to the referees at the score table and let them know I have diabetes. They write diabetes right by my name just in case I get low (or have a problem) on the court.

–Valerie Kintz, age 15

Tip: Test before and after games and mid-game if you feel low.

–Laura Reichstadt, age 14

Tip: When I play pickup games of basketball, I always bring a bunch of snacks and eat between games. All my friends know I have diabetes, but I still have to remind them not to eat my snacks every time we play.

–Herbert Larkin, age 17

Rowing

Julia Halprin Jackson, a student at the University of California, Santa Barbara, was rowing competitively less than a week after being diagnosed. She never let it get her down. She just dealt with it, plain and simple, and has been giving us tips since the day we met.

Julia: Being on the rowing team means 2-hour practices five days a week, and at least one race per weekend. Rowing requires an intense, concentrated effort that goes beyond just working out. A certain mental focus is needed to get the oar into the water at just the right angle, follow other rowers in the boat, listen to commands from the coxswain, and pull with power.

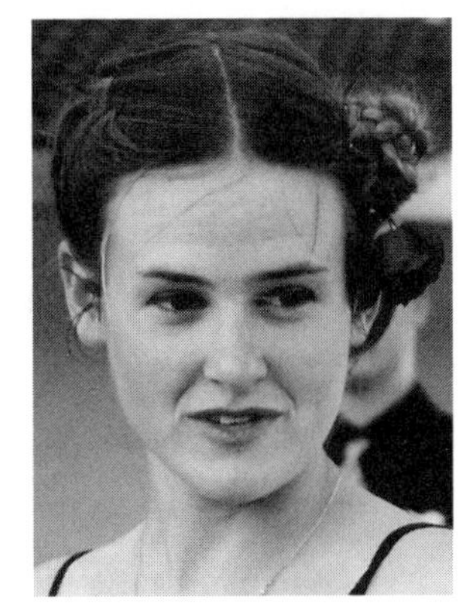

Julia Halprin Jackson

Our typical practice consists of rowing back and forth at the Port, a minimum of a half-mile from the dock, usually a few miles down the river. My coach follows us in a motorboat and shouts commands. Aside from occasional water breaks, we row continuously.

Rowing routine

In the first few days of practice after being diagnosed, I discovered that my blood sugar could drop anywhere from 50 and 100 points at practice, depending on our workout. I was terrified of getting low out on the water.

I found that the best routine for me is to "front-load" about an hour before practice. I eat at least 30 grams of carbohydrate before I leave my house, then test as soon as I get to the Port. If my sugar is less than 130–140, I drink a juice. Ideally, I go out on the water at about 160 or 170. I always make sure to ask my coach how intense a practice to expect, so I can decide how much I want to eat beforehand. No matter what my blood sugar is before the workout, I always take at least two small juice cans for my coxswain to hold during practice. My coach carries my kit with my blood glucose monitor, glucagon, juice, candy, and cell phone in his launch.

Generally I drink one juice before we leave the dock, row for the first hour or so, then drink another during a water break, then test as soon as we get off the water.

I always write down my blood sugars, so I can compare how much the rowing affects my numbers. This was particularly helpful when I was newly diagnosed, because I was still "honeymooning" and learning how much to eat when I rowed.

➡ **Note:** Honeymooning is a period of time—usually a few months to a year—right after diagnosis when your body is still making some insulin.

Insulin Dosage Adjustments While Rowing Competitively

I was diagnosed during the weekend and missed a total of five days of rowing because of diabetes. When I met the endocrinologist in the hospital, I told him how active I planned to be. He took that into consideration when figuring my insulin dosages of Humalog and NPH. He taught my family and me how to adjust the amounts when I had rowing regattas, row-a-thons, or other big events.

I found that my dosage for regattas did not differ much from regular practice days because each race lasted only 7 or 8 minutes, whereas a practice was at least 1–2 hours. I did have some problems with queasiness during races because I drank so much juice beforehand, so it was helpful for me to front-load a few hours before the race or to decrease my pre-race insulin dosages. It was not uncommon for races to be delayed, so I had to be careful during regattas and be open to changes in my routine.

- Bring your kit and cooler to the boathouse.
- Test before an event. I always go into competition with blood sugar at least 170–180.
- Take juice or sports drink and frosting on the boat.
- Reduce insulin after an all-day competition.

The transition at the end of the season affected my blood sugars considerably. I was so exhausted after the nine-month season, on top of high school and diabetes, that by summer, I was ready for a less intense exercise regimen. I increased my insulin dosages because I was exercising less over the summer.

–Julia Halprin Jackson, age 17

Running

Stacy: When I ran cross-country in high school, I drank Propel to keep from going low. Some people dilute Gatorade, so it has fewer carbs to drink while training. We always ran in groups of three or more. That way if someone suffered heat exhaustion, sprained an ankle, or needed help, one person stayed with the runner who was down while the third went for help.

During training I kept my Gatorade, meter, and a tube of glucose or frosting in my athletic bag on the field. My coach also kept juice and Gatorade for me. If I was having a rough day, I'd carry a tube of frosting during workouts. Half an hour after a race, I would drink 8 oz of Gatorade.

- Use powdered Gatorade and mix it with water to the strength you need for various sports.
- I carry a tube of cake decorating frosting in my sock while working out.

–Stacy Gemmell, age 19

Soccer

Eric Brin plays soccer—it's what he loves to do. In high school he played center midfielder. In his freshman year at Northwestern University, his coach moved him to a forward position. Not a bad move considering Eric scored the first goal of the season for the Northwestern Wildcats!

Eric: When the team travels, I stock up on extra snacks and carry them in my athletic bag. When the team travels to away sports tournaments, I *always* get up and have breakfast even if my teammates sleep in. Eating breakfast helps me keep on track! At practice, games, and away games, I carry my kit and snacks in my athletic bag. *–Eric Brin, age 18*

Tip: I play soccer and my favorite halftime snacks are popsicles. They cool me off, replace some of the carbs I use up exercising, and also give me fluids.

–Kelly Hrubeniuk, age 10

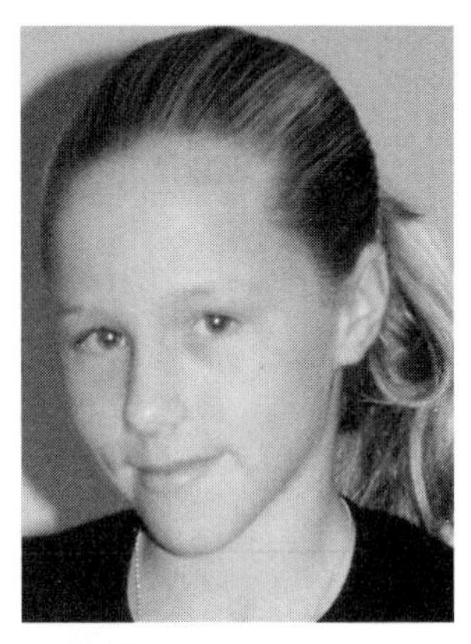

Kelly Hrubeniuk

Tip: Before every soccer game, I test my sugar and drink a little juice.

–Rebecca Parziale, age 9

Tip: When I play soccer, we have a code. When I feel low, I hold up my hand in the shape of an L. Then I come to the sidelines for a drink of Gatorade, or the coach subs me out for a few plays so I can eat.

–Chris Graham, age 11

Water polo and intense pump management

Bo: The former captain of the water polo team at UC Davis, Mary Costello keeps her blood sugar level by lowering her basal rate, testing, and sipping carbs when needed. Her enthusiasm for the pump is catching as she takes pumping and exercise to the next level. I must say, getting to know Mary caused Spike and me to start thinking seriously about the pump.

Mary: I played intercollegiate water polo for the University of California, Davis, for 2 years and now play on the Club Aggie team. It's been tough figuring out how to have good sugar levels during such intense exercise, but I've learned a lot and hope some of it might be useful to you.

I love the pump! I have found a ton of little helpful diabetes tips on www.insulin-pumpers.org. This website is so amazing and supportive. My pump and the support of other insulin pumpers have combined to make my life, my A1C, and my overall health so much better. (Your A1C is an average of your blood sugars over a 3-month period.)

It took a while to get used to the pump, and I had some frustrating episodes the first year. (Watch out for ketones sneaking up on you if your tubing kinks up!) It also took me a while to get used to inserting the cannula. However, my diabetes is so much easier to control now, and I have so few lows that the pros of being on the pump far outweigh these little cons.

Gatorade and other equivalent sports drinks have been so important! They keep me hydrated and give me carbs when I need them. Gatorade is fast acting and doesn't hurt my stomach. Plus, everyone else is drinking sports drinks already! I leave a bottle on the side of the pool and drink from it if I feel low, or if the workout is more intense than I predicted. This little precaution really helps me avoid lows.

It's important to help your teammates and coach understand enough about diabetes, so they know what you need and when you need it. At the beginning of each season, I give my coach a letter explaining what to expect and why I will need to get out in the middle of practice for a minute to check my blood sugar and possibly eat or take insulin. Most importantly, I tell him the symptoms and signs of low blood sugar. I also explain that the first two weeks or so involve a lot of adjusting, and that I will likely get low and need to check my blood sugar a lot. I've noticed that my own security with having diabetes helps my team feel comfortable. They have all been very understanding when I need to get out of the water to eat or check my blood sugar.

➡ **Note:** An important concept to remember is that the more insulin there is hanging out in the body, the more you have to eat to prevent lows AND the higher the chance that you will get low.

I try not to eat anything for the 3 hours before I exercise. This is because I use rapid-acting insulin in my pump, and it lasts for 3–4 hours. If I eat and take insulin during the 3 hours before exercise, some of the bolus insulin I used to cover my food will still be in my body during the exercise. This can lead to lows if I didn't eat quite enough for the exercise I am getting (even when that exercise is hours after my last bolus).

Five to 15 minutes before intense exercise, I eat 60–120 grams of carbohydrate, without insulin. I feel better eating on an empty, hungry stomach, not a full one. You want to try to avoid highs that would require insulin during the 3 hours before exercising, and you want less insulin in your body when you exercise. That's why I check 3 hours before exercising—so I can correct sooner and not have to shoot up a bunch or eat a bunch right before exercise. *I treat the 3 hours before exercising as a very critical time for good control during exercise.*

Another technique I use to decrease the amount of insulin in my body during exercise is to lower my background insulin. For pumpers it usually works to decrease the basal to 0–0.2 for 1–2 hours before exercising. Be careful of highs toward the end of your workout and after you've finished! You may need to take a bolus (1–3 units of rapid-acting insulin) towards the end of your workout or take a small amount of insulin in the middle of a workout to offset highs from the decrease in insulin and the increase in carbs. Be very careful of this method though! Get advice from your doctor to avoid lows from the extra insulin!

Depending on the intensity, duration, and type of exercise, I usually eat 15–120 grams of carbohydrate right before exercising. The longer and the more intense your workout, the more fast-acting carbohydrate you need and the bigger decrease in insulin you need. Sometimes exercise that is not aerobic (like weightlifting) may not require any decrease in insulin or only a slight increase in food. But, if it is aerobic in nature, long and intense, you may need up to 120 grams of carbohydrate. I like

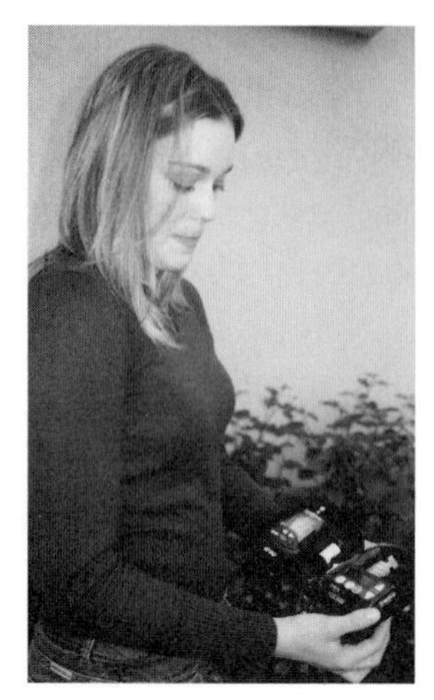

Mary Costello

Jamba Juice smoothies. They have 110–120 grams of carbohydrate, are fast acting, have little protein and fat, and are good for you!

What do you do with your pump if your sport involves water or a lot of contact? I take my pump off during water polo and swimming. If my exercise lasts one hour or longer, I get out of the water half to three-quarters of the way through my workout and take 0.2–1 unit. If I exercise over two hours, I get out of the pool again after two hours and take 1.5–2 units to offset highs from having a decrease in basal for so long. I usually get out one or two times no matter how long a workout is, because I've found taking a little bit of insulin during the workout can help offset highs later on. (I do this by plugging my pump back in and giving a bolus.) Plus I like knowing what my sugars are during a workout.

When your exercise routine changes, so do your insulin needs. If I exercise on a regular basis and then stop for over two days, I have to increase my basal by 0.2. If I stop for over a week, I usually have to increase an additional 0.1–0.2. The injection or infusion site matters too. I've found that if the insulin was injected (or my infusion set is located) somewhere with little body fat, there may be a difference in insulin absorption, and I see more roller coaster sugars. Stick to areas with a little more fat if you notice this trend!

Andy: During water polo "Hell Week" our longest practices last four hours. I like to keep my blood sugar around 160–180 at practice and during games—I would much rather be a little high than crash. I use being a little high as a safety zone. During Hell Week, I discovered I could stay hydrated and also get some

Rule of Thumb

- If I'm high right before exercise and don't have ketones, I can take about one-fourth the insulin I normally take. The exercise will help lower my blood sugar. I always have Gatorade with me, so that I can drink some once my blood sugar is normal. This helps me avoid lows.
- When you are exercising, drinking Gatorade or the equivalent keeps you hydrated and doesn't give you a stomachache.
- When I exercise I get lower faster and more often, and when I'm sedentary I get higher.
- Warm-up, warm-down, and stretching are important for the long-term health of people with diabetes! Try to do all three for every workout.
- Insulin pens are great for water sports. Sometimes I'd get cold waiting for my pump to click in one unit at a time, or I might not have time to wait in the middle of the game. Pens are also good around the pool if your pump isn't water resistant.
- Visit the Diabetes Exercise and Sports Association at www.diabetes-exercise.org. for information on diabetes and exercise.
- *The Diabetic Athlete, Prescriptions for Exercise and Sports* by Sheri Colberg, is an amazing book and gives guidelines for individual sports. For example, you can look up swimming, water polo, weight training, triathlons, and tons more!

–Mary Costello, age 21

carbs by sipping powdered Gatorade diluted in water, throughout practice. I figured out what ratio of powdered Gatorade to water I needed through trial and error.

–Andy Savage, age 15

Sports Tournaments

Sports tournaments entail strenuous exercise for longer periods of time—plus there is the excitement of competition. After strenuous exercise, your warm muscles will take up glucose (sugar) for hours, which means you require less insulin following heavy exercise. *Blood sugar can run low 12 hours, or even 24 hours, after strenuous exercise.* Keep that in mind when you take your evening and nighttime insulin. You will probably need to lower those doses. Pumpers may need to lower their nighttime basal rates after tournament-level exercise.

Tip: Lower your short-acting insulin before heavy exercise, tournaments, competitions, and games. I end up lowering my dose to 1/2 or 1/4 of my normal amount.

–Ant Engeln, age 14

Tip: Test often during all-day sports events.

–Blair Ryan, age 16

Tip: Snack often during all-day sports events. Gatorade, peanut butter and jelly sandwich, whatever you like to eat.

–Rory Tarbox, age 19

Tip: Have a before-bed snack of carbohydrates and protein after a day of heavy exercise.

–Christian Cooper, age 10

Cheerleading

Mollie has been a competitive cheerleader for 9 years—5 years with a dance studio, 3 years in middle school (her all-star years). This is her first year cheering for her high school.

Mollie: In cheerleading competitions we have 4 minutes to do our whole routine, so it's not that difficult to manage. I test two or more times during the hour before a game to make sure I'll have good control. If I am around 100–120, which is normally right where I like to be, I eat 15–20 carbs because I am going to burn a lot of calories during the first half. At halftime I snack again if I am still below 120. My coach is great. She always keeps juice for me in the team ice chest!

- The key to doing all this is to be organized and to stay on top of it. Even if you have to sacrifice doing one cheer or one stunt, it's better to stop and test than risk getting low out on the field.
- If you feel bad, don't think, "I'm letting my team down." Step off the field, check yourself, and drink some juice.
- My favorite quick carb snacks are small cereal bars.

–Mollie Meggs, age 14

Racquetball

Bo: Since coming to USC, racquetball is my new thing. Like many other strenuous sports, racquetball takes a lot of energy, and that means you have to carb up before you play. If I am going to play only one or two games, I try to start with my blood sugar between 120–140. (Here is how I handled racquetball on injections. See page 199 for racquetball on the pump.)

- Always err on the side of caution. Let your sugars go a little higher if it's one of those days when you don't have great control. It is better to start playing at 180 than to start playing at 60.

When I first began to play racquetball 4 years ago, I did the groundwork. I tested my blood after every game and experimented with drinking a little more or less Gatorade and eating either one or two Snickers bars after each game, until I figured out what worked for me.

When my sugar is at 120 before my first game, I drink about 8 oz of Gatorade and eat a fun-size Snickers bar. This provides enough carbs to last 20 minutes or so for the first game. If I know I am going to play a whole series of games, like in a competition, I usually drink a few more sips of Gatorade—plus I bring two 32 oz bottles of Gatorade and four or five fun-size Snickers bars to the court.

After game one, I have a few sips of Gatorade. If I feel well, then I go right into my next game. After I finish with the games, I drink some more Gatorade and go looking for real food. Hopefully, it's dinnertime! After an hour or so of racquetball (four games), even if I drank too much Gatorade and my blood sugar is at 180, because my body has been worked so hard, within a half-hour, my sugars are going to fall about 60 points. If, when I leave the court, I test at 120, then I need to be sure to eat enough carbs to account for the fact that my sugars are going to fall by those 60 points.

Just as with most strenuous activities, if I play more than an hour of racquetball after 6:00 PM, I need to lower my nighttime insulin dose (my Ultra Lente from 18 units to 14 units, or my basal rate from 1.0 to 0.8).

Wrestling tournaments

Rollie: During a daylong tournament, you only have a few matches at 6 minutes apiece, with several hour rests in between. For each match, I pack a cooler with lunch, dinner, snacks, plenty of water, and Gatorade. Wrestlers are notified 30 minutes to an hour before their next match, so there's plenty of time to test and load up on Gatorade if needed.

Wrestling practice is very challenging. Our practices were 3 hours, Monday through Friday, plus an hour of running afterwards. The practices were for conditioning and to build up stamina, so we were working out and sweating for 3 hours straight. *This kind of intense exercise lowers your blood sugar a lot and quickly.*

My original way of handling this was to eat a lot for lunch and to go into practice pretty high (with food on board). I'd usually come out of practice 3 hours later in the 60s. My newer method is to go into practice in the high 100s, having eaten lots of long-lasting foods during the afternoon, and then sip 32 oz of Gatorade all through practice. This worked out better, and I'd come out of practice in the 60–100 range. I'd have additional Gatorade before I went running.

- I prefer Gatorade to juices because the juices sit like a lump in my stomach.
- After a day of heavy exercise, test often and watch your sugars. You may need to lower your nighttime insulin dose to compensate for all the exercise.

–Rollie Berry, age 18

Distance running fine tuned on the pump

Rollie manages wrestling tournaments on injections. Blair has taken controlling her sugars during distance running down to a science. Each method requires different management skills, and both methods work. Blair Ryan is a varsity runner at Ventura High School. She's pumping with a Paradigm.

Blair: We thought that something might have been wrong after my horrible race at the California Interscholastic Federation (CIF) Finals, where I was number 120 out of 123 runners. I had run 2 1/2 minutes slower than on the same course earlier in the season, where I placed 8th out of 200 freshmen. That, combined with my other classic symptoms, pushed us to test for diabetes. Sure enough, I was diagnosed three days before the California State meet in 2000.

Since that day I have run the 800 and the 4 × 400 relay in the CIF Southern Section Prelims, have been on many record-breaking relay teams, and competed all over California. I am on most of the top 25 all-time school performances for cross-country courses, and I ran at the cross-country California State Championships in 2001.

- Remember, with a good attitude, diabetes can't stop you from accomplishing *anything*.

None of these achievements came easily. Distance running is demanding because there are no immediate successes, which also means no shortcuts. You have to be able to look down the road and work toward goals that are months and years away. Because of these qualities, distance runners are a unique group of people. My teammates are my absolute best friends. They helped me make it through the first few months after my diagnosis, as well as through every practice since.

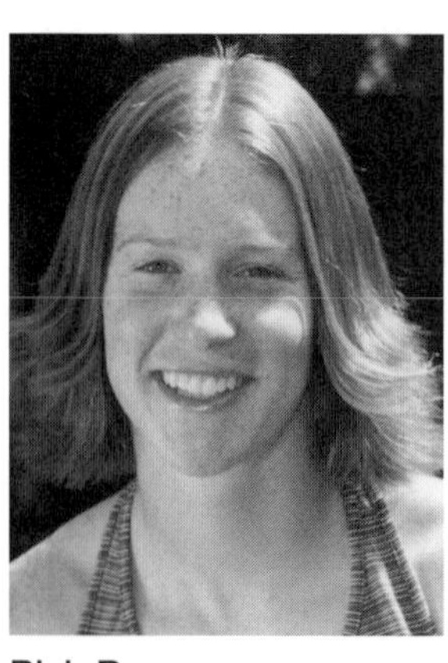

Blair Ryan

- Include your friends and teammates in your diabetes treatment, and they will be more than willing to help.

There are so many things that go into distance running: hydration, food intake, interval work, long aerobic runs, endurance runs, tempo runs, water workouts—and the list goes on. Now when you add blood sugars, adrenaline, basal rates, meal coverage, glycogen stores, morning workouts, afternoon workouts, evening workouts, and replenishment on top of that, it gets a little complicated.

Every practice for me is another trial and error. No two practices are exactly alike. Because of this, I have had several meetings with my diabetes specialist to really nail down a routine that works for me.

- It is important to get advice from a doctor or other diabetes specialist on handling your diabetes during strenuous activities like competitive running. It is especially important when you are having a tough time controlling your sugars or are experiencing too much fatigue or stiffness.

Long distance day (serious mileage)

My routine varies depending on the type of running I will be doing. I aim for a blood sugar of 200 pre-workout. I get my sugar up to 200 by under-covering my lunch: 1 unit to every 1 1/2 carbs (22 grams carbohydrate) instead of my usual 1 to 1 (1 unit of insulin to 15 grams carbohydrate). (No, it is not the best to have it high, but it isn't high that long, and the run brings it down. All of my A1Cs have been between 5.4 and 6.5.) If I have eaten some long-acting carbs, my blood sugar usually sustains on a non-stop run. I have sewn pockets into my running shorts and have at least two 15-carb glucose tablets with me every run.

- Sew pockets into your running shorts to keep glucose tablets with you on long distance runs.

If I feel low on a run, I stop and eat the carbs. If I am lower than I want before the run, I drink Ultra Fuel by Twin Lab. This drink has a concentration of 99 grams of carbohydrate in 16 oz (roughly 6 1/2 carbs per oz). This has been the best thing I've tried because it is not like eating the chalky tablets, and the texture of bars grosses me out. Ultra Fuel makes correcting lows really fast. Many times before a workout, I have had to drink two bottles of it because my sugar wouldn't go up. Drinking Ultra Fuel is better than chewing 39 glucose tablets, as I am sure you can imagine. If my blood sugar is too high going into a workout (I consider over 230 to be too high), then I take 0.2 units of fast-acting insulin.

Interval workouts

These workouts are a little more convenient because they are usually around the track, or we come back to the same area between intervals. This gives me access to more than just my pump and the tablets that I store in my homemade pockets.

I feel best if I am running with a blood sugar between 150 and 180. But workouts in particular, and even warm-ups, tend to bring my sugar down dramatically. For interval workouts, I end up drinking Ultra Fuel during warm-up and between intervals. In a workout like this, we may do a 3-mile warm-up, then 6 × 800 meters at 2:56–3:05 pace, then a mile cool-down. I test pre-warm-up, post-warm-up, between the second and third 800s, between the sixth and seventh 800s, and after the cool-down. This is a lot of testing, but it is necessary. My blood sugars fluctuate so quickly that I might need to drink more Ultra Fuel during the 2 minutes before the next interval (when I am below 150) or take a 0.1 unit bolus (if I am above 180).

While stretching after workouts, my team and I replenish with a Power Bar, Luna Bar, or other substantial food or drink.

Race day

- Before a race I eat a whole-grain bagel with peanut butter. These long-acting carbs are stored as energy that I'll need later.

My coach and I have made my main goal for warm-up on race day getting my sugar to 150 on the starting line, while doing as much of the warm-up with my team as I can. We do the 3-mile course once when we first get to a meet. At that time I want my sugar about 140. These three miles are low intensity. When we are done with that, we usually have a little time before our actual warm-up. During this time I test about four times, because on race days adrenaline is sort of my enemy. The more nervous I am the more my sugar creeps up. I constantly give 1-unit boluses to bring my sugar down into the 150 area. Then, 35 minutes before we need to be on the starting line, we do the second part of the warm-up—10 minutes of running and drills. After these I test again. If the adrenaline is not having an effect and my sugar is below 150, I stop and drink Ultra Fuel. If my sugar is high from the adrenaline, then I take a bolus and do the cut-down run and strides. I would bolus one unit for every 40 points my blood sugar is above 150.

Once on the starting line, I take a bolus to cover the adrenaline that shoots glucose into my blood throughout the intensity of the race. If my sugar is 150, then I'll take 1.5 units on the line. I'll take more if it is higher (2.5 units if it is 230). After I have taken my bolus, I detach the pump and hand it to my parents, coach, or a non-racing teammate. After that, it is me, my teammates, and the course!

- Test a lot between warm-ups and race time. The better your sugars are when you start, the better your place at the finish.
- Since the pump can bounce when running, my mom and I invented a Velcro strap that is better than those we could buy. It keeps my pump close to my body so that there is no distracting bouncing. It is just a simple elastic strap, 1 inch wide with Velcro on both ends. I put the strap under my shorts' elastic waistline. The strap goes under the pump clip, so that the pump is between the strap and me.
- The infusion site of the pump still scares me, but I feel it is better to have to insert it every 3 days than to take 6 shots a day. I use Emla cream (it numbs the skin a little). Forty-five minutes before I am going to replace the infusion site, I put a quarter-size glob of Emla cream on my skin and then cover it with Tegaderm Transparent Dressing. I can even shower while it is on. Now there have been many times where it has not been convenient to use it, and I have done fine without it, but it is nice to have.

–Blair Ryan, age 16

Be Prepared for Anything

River mouth at Dominical, Costa Rica

What started out as a beautiful day of surfing in Costa Rica turned into a search and rescue. When disaster struck, Spike and I had everything we needed in our coolers on shore and were able to join the rescue effort without missing a beat.

Bo: It was another beautiful day in Dominical. Standing on the shore, snacking from the stash in my cooler, I was reminiscing about the absolutely perfect wave I had caught only half an hour earlier. It was the clean-up wave. I sensed it coming as it rose up behind me and began to break ten feet to my right. I paddled once, popped up, dropped in, and tried to get tubed. The wave crested and was hitting the back of my board. I got barreled. After a good bottom turn, I went up for a slice on top, tried to pull a floater but didn't make it. Rode the wave in on my belly, cheering the whole way.

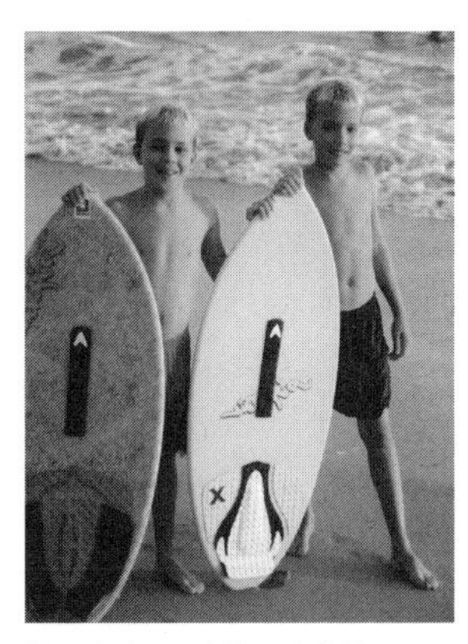

Derrick and Daniel Crowe

Back on shore, relaxed, satisfied and finishing a snack from my cooler, I thought I'd like to catch one more wave. The paddle out was easy this time because I went right after another cleanup set. Duck-diving one big wave I got stung by broken-off jellyfish tentacles. It happens. There was a real crowd on the lineup now. I didn't think I was going to get another wave. Then I noticed the commotion outside.

A longboarder was paddling furiously out to where the river spewed into the ocean. In front of the longboarder, about a hundred yards out, there was a kid frantically thrashing his hands in the water. Spike, Ryan, Erik, and I, and all the other surfers in the water, started paddling after the longboarder, towards the kid. We all arrived where the boy went under at the same time. Now everyone was off their boards, leashes on their ankles, diving, trying to find the kid.

After what seemed like an eternity, the longboarder came up with the boy and dragged him onto his board. The kid was puking water and shrieking. Exhausted, the longboarder placed the kid on his board and started the long paddle in. I paddled alongside, pushing the back of his board. When we got to the whitewater, I rode in fast to ditch my board and then went back to help the longboarder steady his board. The kid was rigid, his hands clamped to the side of the board. After we laid him on the sand, we gave the rescued boy some of our Gatorade to help calm him down. He was talking now.

He and his little brother had been playing in the river. They hadn't realized how swift the current was after last night's rain. He lost his footing and was swept out into the ocean where he was trapped in a terrible rip tide, in the white water where the big surf was breaking and the river water was flowing out to sea. The kid panicked and was going under when the longboarder saved him.

- Being organized and prepared sometimes benefits others in unexpected ways.

Backpacking and the great outdoors

With foresight and careful planning, diabetes can go anywhere. Kelly Hrubeniuk, age 10, has vacationed at the beach and on a houseboat on Lake Powell, taken trips on airplanes, and gone hiking and four wheeling. She recently added backpacking to her adventures, hiking to 9,000 feet and camping in the wilderness for four days.

Kelly: I carried my monitor and supplies in my backpack, and my mom carried a back-up monitor and supplies in hers. With all the hiking and climbing, my blood sugars ran a little on the low side. I checked my sugars twice as often as usual, but I didn't mind. We adjusted my insulin down, and I had a blast!

- Always carry back-up supplies when you are going to be a long way from civilization.
- Ask one of your hiking buddies (or parents) to carry back-up supplies too.

–Kelly Hrubeniuk, age 10

Tip: When I go pheasant hunting with my dad, I keep my cooler filled with snacks in the pickup truck and carry Juicy Juices and granola bars when we hike through the foothills. *–Christian Cooper, age 10*

Snowboarding and Cold Weather

Bo: Spike and I look at cold weather as another thing that drains energy. Your body has to expend energy to exercise and to keep warm. When I spend the same amount of time at the same level of exertion in cold weather (snowboarding versus playing soccer), I eat 30–40% more carbs. When I hit the slopes, instead of eating one fun-size Snickers bar, I might have two. Instead of 8 oz of Gatorade, I might have 12 oz. When you are on the mountain, you are a lot farther away from food than when you are playing soccer, so carry plenty of snacks.

- I carry three full-size candy bars, a small can of juice, and a tube of cake frosting (or glucose gel) in my fanny pack.
- Return to the lodge every hour and a half to eat and test.

Insulin, meters, and pumps are sensitive to the cold, so they need to be kept next to your body. Some meters have to warm up before they work, and if insulin gets too cold, it can be damaged and lose its potency. This causes problems in trying to gauge how much insulin to take.

- Keep your insulin and meter warm. I carry mine in the inside zipper pocket of my jacket, close to my body. If you are on the pump, keep your pump, tubing, and meter insulated and close to your body for warmth.

Cold weather puts an additional stress on your body. It takes calories to keep you warm. You'll eat more food and need to lower your insulin before, during, and after very active cold-weather sports like skiing and snowboarding. When I was on injections I always lowered my nighttime insulin 50% or more after a full day of snowboarding. Pumpers, you may need to lower your nighttime basal rate (page 191).

Tip: Being at high altitude lowers blood sugar.
–Andy Savage, age 15

Tip: When I am on the slopes, I carry granola bars in my pocket, something with substance. When you snowboard—lows happen. *–Andy Savage, age 15*

Scuba-Diving and Cold Water

If you scuba-dive, or try any new sport for that matter, play it safe. Test before, during, and after; eat a lot more calories than usual; and definitely, take a cooler with you for all the extra food that you will need.

Bo: The diving books warn people with diabetes to beware of SCUBA (Self Contained Underwater Breathing Apparatus). My motto has always been that you should let nothing get in your way, especially something as controllable as diabetes. With that in mind, I decided to take a scuba certification course here in Ventura.

I found that, just as in any other extreme sport, if you are well-organized, it's no big deal. If you account for the energy expenditure and the calorie intake, then you've got it covered. When it was time for my first dive, I checked my sugar, and it was 140. This is normally right where I like to keep my sugars before hard exercise. Because I wasn't sure what to expect from scuba, I drank 10 oz of Gatorade and ate a bite-size Snickers.

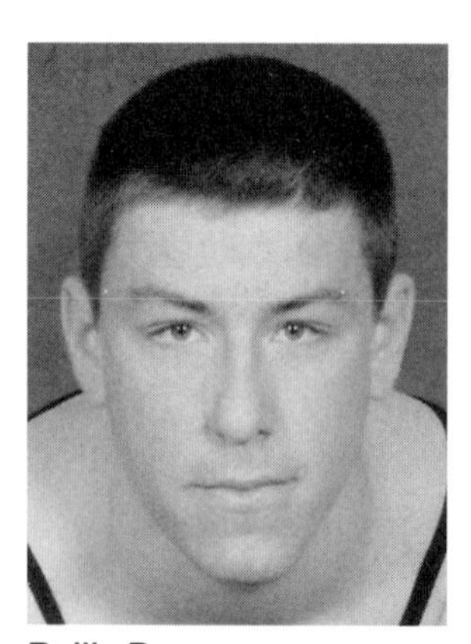

Rollie Berry

While my instructor walked over to the edge of the boat (about 10 feet off the water) and jumped in, I finished putting on the last of my gear, put my goggles on my face, and pulled my fins onto my feet. Before I jumped in, I filled my Buoyancy Control Device (BCD) to make sure I didn't sink with the weight of all the gear. When it was my turn, I walked over to the edge and took a "giant's stride" into the water. When the last person was in the water, my instructor signaled for us to descend. It was awesome! The feeling of weightlessness, total freedom, and the pure excitement of being able to breathe under water was exhilarating. When I surfaced and came off the high of seeing crabs, sea lions, Garibaldi, and all sorts of other cool underwater life, I realized that the essentials of scuba diving boiled down to a few things.

- Cold water causes your body to burn calories faster than normal. The deeper the dive, the colder the water, the faster your body burns carbs.
- Breathing out of a scuba tank takes more effort than breathing at the surface, which again causes your body to burn calories at an accelerated rate.

Whenever you do anything for the first time, in particular something that can be frightening, like being 70 feet underwater, the new experience can excite you to such a point that you use up your energy faster than you might expect.

- Test your blood sugar before tackling a new sport.
- Get to know what balance of insulin and calories is required for every sporting activity.
- Take your cooler on the dive boat. If you're diving from shore, make sure you put your food in a cooler on the beach, so animals can't get into it or drag it off.

Tip: When you scuba, test an hour before, half an hour before, and right before a dive to see *where your blood* *sugar is trending*. If it is low or heading down, eat something with sugar and carbs. My blood sugar is better when I dive than at any other time because I monitor myself so closely. I also carry glucose-gel in my buoyancy control device (BC-vest). *–Clare Rosenfeld, age 16*

Tip: Pumpers: No matter how comfortable you feel, strip down your wetsuit, and check your insertion site after every dive. *–Clare Rosenfeld, age 16*

Rollie: It was pretty exciting going diving for the first time in Fiji. I had no idea what to expect, so I tested before each dive and tried to be about 150 when I went in the water. The dive crew had thermoses of juice on the dive boat for washing the salt-water taste out of your mouth, so I had access to fresh juice, but I never needed it. I kept glucose gel in my board shorts under my wetsuit. I don't know how much good that would have done, but it made my mother happy. They were easy dives, about 45 minutes each. I found that 45 minutes of easy underwater exploration lowered my blood sugar about 75 points.

- At scuba class, I learned (after falling into the water) that glucose tablets in the little plastic tube melt immediately in your pocket and make a gooey mess.
- Keep your kit and snacks safe on the beach or boat when you are scuba-diving, surfing, snorkeling, skimboarding, swimming, bodysurfing, doing anything in the water.

–Rollie Berry, age 18

Bo and the Seagulls

On a recent trip to Baja, where the water is really warm and the surf is incredible, we felt like hardened surf veterans who could handle anything Baja threw our way. We had already dealt with some kind of Central American crocodile, been stung by a few jellyfish, and managed to live through some really big waves at Playa Negra. We never thought seagulls would present the biggest challenge on our surf adventure.

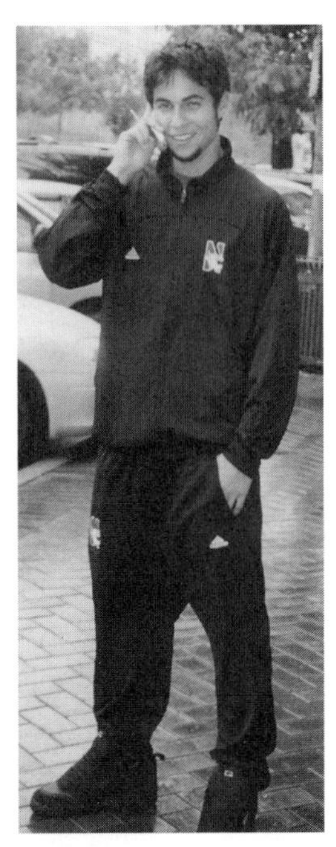
Eric Brin

Bo: The surf was good, 6 foot and glassy, with a little offshore wind, so you can imagine that when I got out there, I didn't want to come in and miss any surf. My brother and I, our three best friends, and all our parents were out surfing at Nine Palms. After about an hour and a half, Spike and I went in to snack up. We grabbed a granola bar and some Gatorade and were back out in the surf in no time. Another hour of riding perfect waves went by. The parents were getting tired and headed in for an afternoon break. As they were paddling in, I heard some commotion, and then howling laughter. To my dismay, a dozen seagulls had gotten into our food. (Spike must have left the cooler open.) They were having a veritable seagull beach party.

A big gull had one of our granola bars in his mouth. Another was munching on our beef jerky and still others were feasting on our chips. We started paddling in and yelling at the gulls, when one big bird lifted off with a battered bag of Doritos in its beak. As he flew away, he sprinkled our snack up and down the beach. A whole team of his friends was right behind him, scouring the sand and devouring every morsel he dropped. The gulls were so intent on taking all of our food that one was even pecking away at a 32 oz bottle of Gatorade. Luckily, it was too heavy, and he left it for us.

- Watch out for seagulls.
- Keep your food in a cooler on the beach with the lid closed to keep it safe from birds and dogs.
- Put your insulin or pump (in a sealable plastic bag) inside your cooler and put it in the shade or at least under a beach towel to help keep it cool.
- Put a couple of ice packs in your cooler so your insulin stays cool.

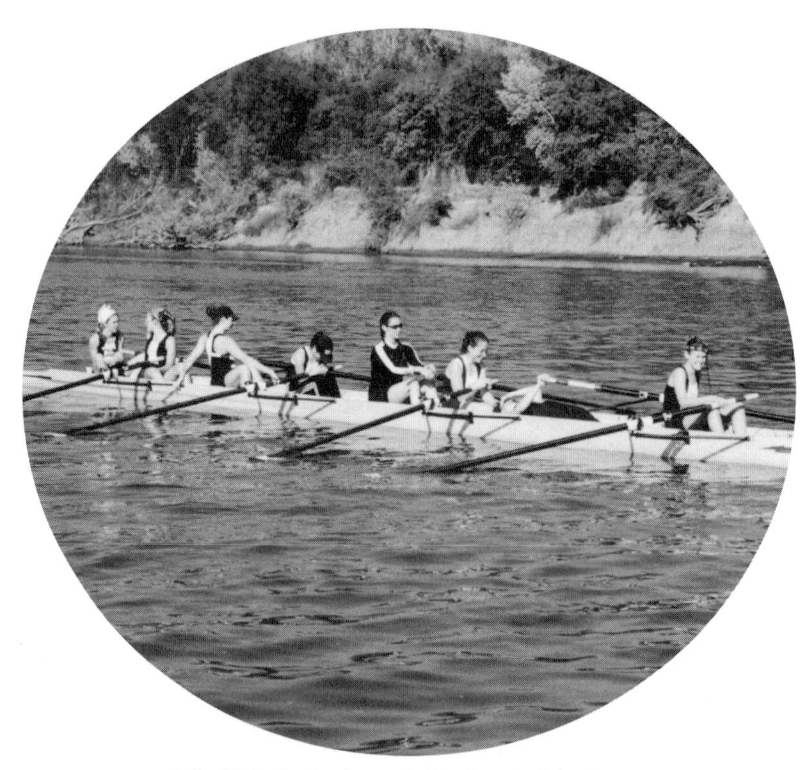

Julia Halprin Jackson in the front of the boat.

CHAPTER THREE

Off to School

Preschool Know-How and Toddlers

Bo: Toddlers need to be tested often. Ryan Kelson's mom and dad test Ryan 5 or 6 times a day and at midnight. Ryan is 2 1/2 years old. He shows no signs when he is low, but when he's high, he sometimes acts out of sorts or angry. It may take years for toddlers to recognize that they are low and to learn to communicate it to their folks.

That's why toddlers need to be tested often!

We saw this tip on the net. It's a verbal check to see if it is time to test.

Tip: Teach toddlers a nursery rhyme and repeat it often. When you suspect low blood sugar, ask them to repeat the well-known rhyme. If little kids get confused repeating the rhyme, it's a good bet they have low blood sugar.

We have known Laura Valine since she was two years old. "Princess" Laura is five now. She is just beginning to realize when she is feeling low and communicate it to her mom and dad. Her folks say she gets better at recognizing low blood sugars all the time.

Tip: I know when I am low because I fall down.

–Laura Valine, age 5

Laura uses exercise to help keep her sugars level—ballet, soccer, swimming and, of course, playing with her friends.

Laura: I like to swim and dance. I had a mommy-and-me ballet class. It was really funny; my mommy had to do some of the stuff we do. Our ballet teacher asked us to help our moms do stuff like a *grand plie*. I told my mom, "Do it like this Mom, pick up the balloon and let it go."

Laura has an imaginary friend, Lennie, who has diabetes. Lennie has brothers and sisters, and sometimes, they all need snacks and drinks and places set at the table. Laura also has a stuffed doggie named Moonshine who has diabetes. Sometimes Moonshine gets low. Laura knows when Moonshine is low, because he falls down too.

- I have a Low Bucket full of things I like to eat. Kids should have a Low Bucket like mine. When we go to the store and I really want something, I ask my mom, "Can I get this for my low bucket? Can I get a Power Puff Girls' sucker?"
- My favorite snacks are Cheetos, BBQ potato chips, no-sugar fudgesicles, and meat sticks.
- I take my cooler to school every day!

–Laura Valine, age 5

Sara Morda, age 4, began dealing with diabetes when she was three and a half. Her mom, Dawn, says Sara is just beginning to let her know when she is low. When Sara is whiney or cranky, that's usually a sign she is low, so they test and then drink some juice and have a snack. When Sara gets low in the middle of the night, she shrieks. Then her mom gives her some juice.

Tip: When I need to eat I say, "Mommy, I can't walk anymore."

–Sara Morda, age 4

When Anela Okamoto, age 3, reports to her mom and dad that she feels low, they test her. If she's low, she gets a sugary drink. But if her sugar is OK, they give her a no-sugar drink. This helps Anela feel good about reporting to her folks that she feels low while she is still learning to recognize the symptoms. (Strawberry, orange, grape, and kiwi are her favorite flavors.)

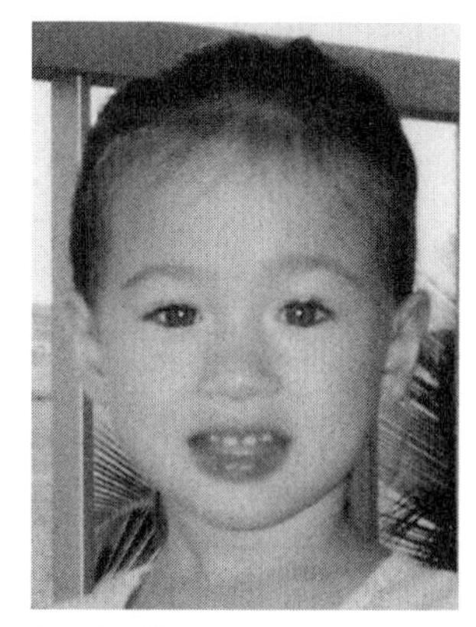

Anela Okamoto

Tip: When I feel low, I say, "Mom, I need something. I need orange juice. My sugar's too low."

–Anela Okamoto, age 3

Sarah Dorsey is three years old. She was diagnosed at 20 months and was the first little kid put on the pump at CHOC (Children's Hospital Orange County).

Any time Sara goes to her mom out of the blue and says, "Mommy, I'm hungry," it's usually a sign that she is pretty low, and her mom tests her right away.

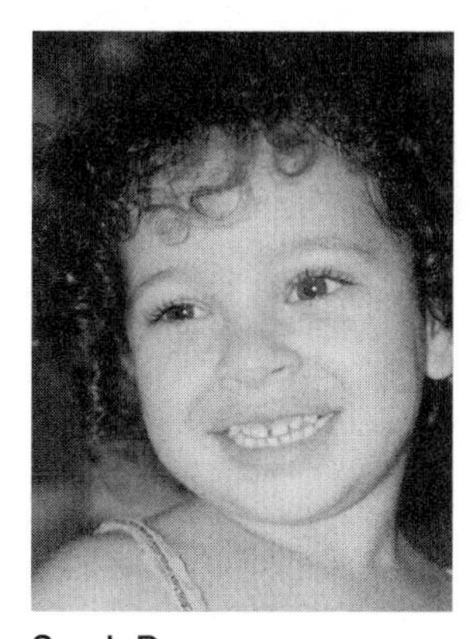

Sarah Dorsey

Tip: My meter is my best friend. (Sarah's mom helped her give this tip.)

–Sarah Dorsey, age 3

Tip: I use the FreeStyle on my arm or leg because it uses a little blood! *–Trey Darensbourg, age 4*

Some toddlers stir their food around on their plate (Bo used to put his cereal bowl on his head), feed their breakfast to the dog, or eat a lot one morning and nothing the next. If you're not sure what your toddler is going to eat for breakfast, eat first and then inject insulin to cover the carbs after breakfast.

Tip: In the morning I eat breakfast, then have my shot.
–Marissa Williams, age 4

Tip: When Marissa feels low, she tells her mom, "Mom, I feel tired." *–Marissa Williams, age 4*

Tip: Mom says diabetes is like brushing your teeth. This is the way it is, and then we just do it.
–Marissa Williams, age 4

Tip: When Jordan feels low, she says, "Mom, I feel yucky."
–Jordan White, age 4

Cameron Olson's mom was also his preschool teacher. They incorporated Cameron's blood test into the "circle" before lunch. All the kids at preschool watched and were interested. Every day before lunch the two- and three-year-old kids would say, "Cameron, it's time to test your blood."

Tip: I keep my supplies in my backpack.
–Cameron Olson, age 5

Tip: When Cameron is low, he says, "Mom, I'm hungry," or "Mom, I'm starting to fall down. I think I'm low."
–Cameron Olson, age 5

Grade School

Have your mom and dad go to your school and talk to your teachers before the first day of school, and let all of your teachers know about your diabetes. Your parents should tell them about your symptoms of highs and lows, what to do in case you get low, and that you should never have to take a quiz or test when you are low.

Spike: We always kept special food at the school. Bo and I each had our own cooler full of snacks and caramels for lows with us every day. In addition to that we kept fully packed coolers under our teacher's desk and in the office. If you have a nurse's office, you could keep one there, too.

Let all of your friends know about diabetes and teach them about it. Our friends helped us out all the time in grade school. Sometimes they would come with us to the office, sometimes they would carry some extra food for us on field trips, and sometimes they would ask us if we were low before we even knew it ourselves!

Tip: It's a good idea to have your mom or dad go to school on the first day and read *Taking Diabetes To School* to your class. Just change the name to yours. Then have a question and answer time to get all the curiosity over with. Check your blood sugar and show them your site, so they won't want to watch you all year.

–Natalie Bayne, age 10

Tip: Keep Diet Coke in the classroom. That way when the other kids get treats and special birthday snacks, you can have a bite of the cupcake and a Coke.

–Brittany Rausch, age 15

Tip: I take my lunch to school, so I know what I am eating.

–Rebecca Parziale, age 9

Tip: I go to a small school. I take the lunch my mom makes to school in my cooler. At lunch I test. Then I go to the cafeteria, and they microwave my lunch.

–David Ashby, age 6

Tip: Tell the bus driver and substitute bus drivers that you have diabetes. When I was in kindergarten, we made up a little flyer with my picture that said: Kenna has diabetes. If she acts funny or says, "I'm dreaming," give her some juice from her backpack. The school bus driver put one on the visor of the bus. *–Kenna Connell, age 16*

Tip: I was diagnosed when I was 9 years old, so when I was in grade school, I told my whole class about diabetes. The kids asked all kinds of questions. They wanted to know how to help. I told them that if I got low I needed some sugar fast and that there was juice in the office. They also knew that if I passed out they should get help and that my glucagon kit was in the health office.

–Laura Reichstadt, age 14

Tip: Tell the kids you hang out with what to do if you get low. *–Laura Reichstadt, age 14*

Tip: Sometimes kids in your class who don't know a lot about diabetes might think it's not fair when you get to eat in class. My teacher just tells them they are welcome to have a snack if they'll check their blood sugar like I do. This usually turns them into one of your best friends because they see what you do every day.

–Natalie Bayne, age 10

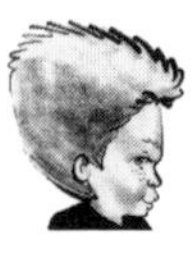

Wish we had thought of that one when we were in grade school.

Jake Burnett and Michael Stratton have been best friends since their first day of preschool. They don't remember life without each other, and since Jake was only four when diagnosed, they don't remember life without diabetes either. Michael is Jake's greatest asset. He reads labels and counts carbs with Jake. Jake and Michael go to the school office every day before lunch to have Jake's blood tested. They check (with the school secretary supervising), play a game of guessing what the number will be, then return to have lunch together. Michael was even given a "Special Friend" award at the end of the school year.

Not all adults know about diabetes. You can help explain things to them, but if they say you're not allowed to eat and you need to eat, go ahead and eat anyway. Your mom or dad can explain to them later why you ate.

Tip: For field trips, walks, etc., I wear a fanny pack with a bottle of glucose tablets, monitor kit, and a bottle of water.
–Benjamin Siegel, age 7

Tip: I didn't let diabetes hold me back. I skipped 6th grade!
–Chris Graham, age 12

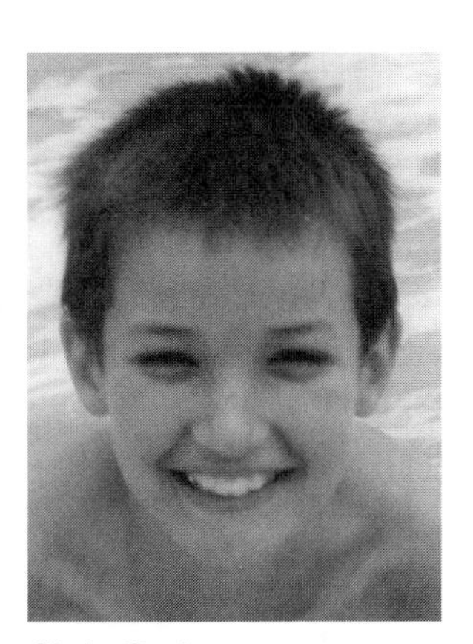

Chris Graham

What a difference a day makes

Spike: I was a real good student all through elementary school. My report cards were full of O's for Outstanding—except sometimes for "Shares well with peers," in which I'd occasionally get the old N for Needs Improvement, but that's another story. I did all my homework and did well on just about every test. I say just about because I remember one test in particular that was really bad.

The day started like any other. I woke up, got dressed, tested and shot up and ate a plate full of toast, bacon, and eggs. I had milk *and* orange juice that morning because I was a little low. Instead of watching a few minutes of GI Joe like I normally did when I was ready to go to school early, I looked over my history packet to try and learn a few more things for my test on the Thirteen Colonies that morning in social studies. My mom helped me.

"Massachusetts?" she asked

"Boston." I replied. That was such an easy one.

"New York?"

"Albany." That one was tricky. I always thought the capital of New York should be New York. Those crazy colonists.

She asked a few more, and I answered right a few more times.

"How about Florida?"

"Mommm! That wasn't even one of the Thirteen Colonies!"

"Oh yeah, I knew that. Right, well, you know the capitals of all the colonies. Let's go to school." (I think she was embarrassed.)

After our morning reading and a short break we finally took our test. When Mr. Scofield put mine in front of me, I just stared at it. For some weird reason, I couldn't think of a single answer. I saw the word Massachusetts but didn't have a clue in the world what I should write in the blank. I moved on. New Jersey. . . .

I had known the answer yesterday and at breakfast and on the drive to class. (I made my mom review them one more time with me, so I could be the first one finished with the test.) But now I didn't know the answers. I left that one blank, too. I think I wrote in New York after New York. I knew that wasn't the right answer, but it was my only guess.

After 10 minutes were up, Mr. Scofield came around to collect our tests. When he asked me to hand in mine, I just stared at him and he picked it up off my desk.

"Hmm," he said, "Spike, is something the matter?" I didn't answer. "Maybe we had better call your mother."

Mr. Scofield let the other kids take a break, and we went to the office to call my mom. She got down to the school in a hurry. She immediately fed me a caramel and a granola bar and tested my finger. I was only 35. No wonder I couldn't think of the capital of Delaware. It was amazing that I could even read the word on the page. I stayed in the office eating caramels and drinking juice from my cooler that we kept there, and my mom tested me again 20 minutes later. I was back up to 85 and wanted to go out and play when I heard the recess bell ring. My mom made me stay and eat my whole snack—a banana, some Cheez-its, and string cheese—before she let me go out and play. I only got to play basketball for 5 minutes. She stayed and thanked Mr. Scofield and asked him to let me take the test again. He said "No problem." The next day I stayed in during recess and re-took the test. I got 13 out of 13. He showed me my first one and said I had gotten 0 out of 13. What a difference a day makes!

Now I know that using your brain can use as much energy as using your muscles. Thinking hard is hard work, and you can't do it well if your blood sugar is low, just like you wouldn't play a soccer game with a low blood sugar.

- It is important to let your teachers know that you can't take tests if you are low, and that if you do a really bad job on a

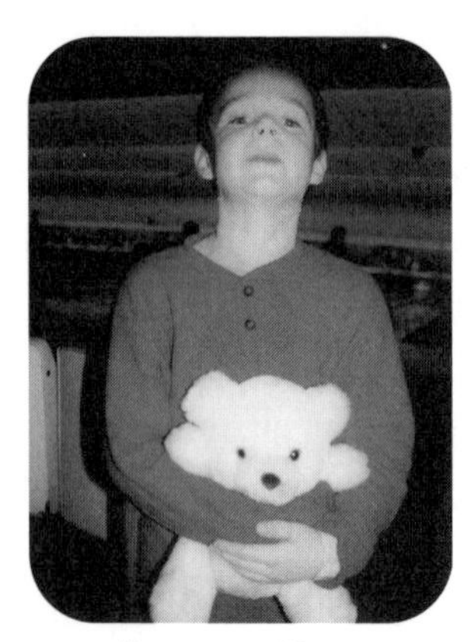
Cameron Olson

test, they should let you retake it. That is if you did badly because of diabetes and not because you didn't study enough.

Ever since that day, even through college, I always have a granola bar and a bottle of Gatorade with me whenever I know I am going to take a test. I sip the Gatorade as I go along and eat the granola bar if the test is long enough for us to take a break. If I ever feel low, of course, I eat the whole thing and follow it up with more food, even if I am right in the middle of a test. If I feel like I need more time, I just tell my teacher that I am having a low sugar and will be unable to finish in the allotted time. I haven't had a problem yet.

Holidays

Christmas morning, Halloween, Chanukah, or the excitement of the Fourth of July can be over-stimulating and cause low blood sugars, especially for young kids. Everyone we ever talked to were low on Christmas morning when they were kids. With this in mind, here are some holiday tips.

Christmas and Chanukah

Tip: Have a big snack containing carbs and protein on Christmas Eve. *–Christian Cooper, age 10*

Tip: Eat breakfast before or during the Christmas morning excitement. I like a big breakfast of bacon, eggs, cheese, and toast. *–Christian Cooper, age 10*

Kids can really get over-stimulated when the family gets together for exciting celebrations like Chanukah and the long Passover meal. Test often and snack frequently.

Halloween

Go ahead and trick-or-treat. You can save some of your favorite bite-sized candy bars for when you are low. Trade the rest of your candy for sugarless gum or money or give it away.

Tip: You'll need a good dinner before going out to trick-or-treat. It's so exciting you can get low.
–Jake Gershenson, age 7

Tip: Take good snacks in your trick-or-treat bag—string cheese, jerky, crackers, and cheese.
–Catilini Ceballos, age 11

Tip: Take your kit. You may need to test.
–Jake Gershenson, age 7

Tip: Don't forget to put yourself on a temporary basal (lower basal by 50%) when you'll be running around during Halloween night. *–Jake Gershenson, age 7*

Tip: Only eat one or two pieces of candy while you're running around trick-or-treating. Save the rest for your cooler. *–Bo*

Tip: I always get low on Halloween, even if I eat some candy. Halloween is exciting! *–Matt DiPaolo, age 12*

Tip: After you go trick-or-treating for Halloween, you can sell your candy to your mom and dad and their friends. I made a bunch of money one year. You can also take some of your candy to the nursing home and the hospital. This makes you feel even better than making money. *–Natalie Bayne, age 10*

Tip: I go trick-or-treating, then save a couple of my favorite candies for lows. My grandpa collects candy, so I give him the rest! *–Catilini Ceballos, age 11*

Tip: I picked two pieces of candy and put my basket in the backyard. The Pumpkin Fairy came and took my candy and left me a Spiderman Web Blaster!
–Carson Canada, age 5

Tip: I check my sugar before I trick-or-treat. I don't eat anything until I get home and show mom.
–Cameron Olson, age 5

Tip: I don't eat any candy when I am out trick-or-treating, but I keep some of my candy for lows and for dessert.
–Khalia Parham, age 10

Tip: I save my favorite trick-or-treat candy for special times and eat it when I am low.
–Kimberly Barkfelt, age 12

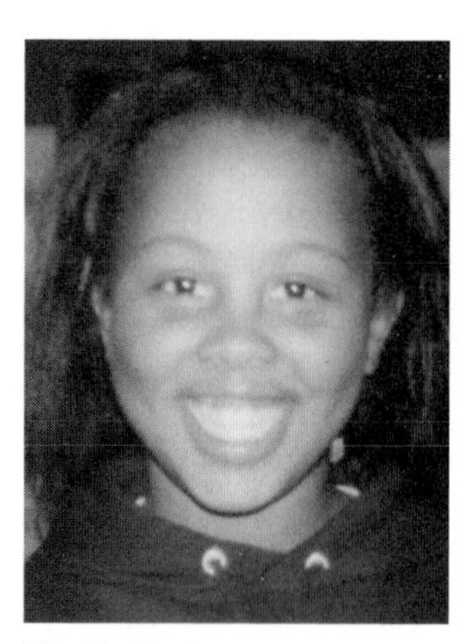

Khalia Parham

The Candy Witch

When Brittany Rausch was diagnosed (at age 2) her folks were worried about how to handle Halloween. Another family told them about the "Candy Witch." The Candy Witch comes on Halloween night and takes all the candy from trick-or-treating and leaves toys or something special in its place. Her parents never linked diabetes to the Candy Witch, but said that she came to save little kids from bad teeth, bad skin, and bad nutrition. They had a special Candy Witch bowl, and their kids got to save 7 pieces of candy (one a day for a week)—the rest went in the bowl. Every Halloween, Brittany's friends got bored with their candy after a few days and then got a little jealous of the gifts left by the Witch. They asked why the Candy Witch didn't come to their house! Happy Trick-or-Treating!

Valentine's Day

When we were in grade school, there was always a classroom party on Valentine's Day full of candy and sweets. Believe it or not, little kids often get so excited at class parties that they eat the cupcake or cookie and still get low. Remember, excitement lowers blood sugar.

- OK it with your teacher, then take a diet soda to drink at the party. The rest of the kids will have to drink that syrupy punch!
- Go ahead and eat the cupcake, but scrape off the frosting first.
- Eat a little protein and fat (nuts, jerky, or cheese) from your cooler along with the cupcake or cookie. You want to feel good so just eat one!

Easter Morning

This is another exciting day for little kids. There is a lot of running around and often a lot of candy to be found!

- Eat breakfast, then hunt for eggs. Better yet, eat a hard-boiled egg and a glass of milk.
- Ask the Easter Bunny for neat things in your basket such as sugarless gum, jerky, GI Joes, a Beanie Baby, or other little things a rabbit can carry.

Bar Mitzvah and Bat Mitzvah

Performing at a long, intense religious service in front of family and friends is both exciting and intellectually stressful. Remember, the brain soaks up glucose like a sponge. Plan your insulin and calories accordingly.

- Lower your insulin or basal before the morning ceremony and have a glass of Gatorade on hand.
- Test often throughout this exciting day!

Indoor Activities

Carry a secret snack into the theatre when attending the opera, a play, or ballet. The same goes for church, temple, and weddings. Try putting a chewy granola bar in your pocket. They aren't messy, and they chew quietly.

Tip: If I need a snack during church, I eat Quaker Oats Cereal Bars. They taste good, and they are soft and quiet.

–Christian Cooper, age 10

Tip: I eat a good breakfast before church. If I get low in church, I eat crackers or a granola bar.

–Catilini Ceballos, age 11

Tip: I carry a box of lemonade in my pocket. If I get low, I drink it.

–Stephen Whitlock, age 16

Tip: If I get low in church, I eat a glucose tablet or a cereal bar or drink a juice.

–Marissa Williams, age 4

Tip: I carry a good snack in my pocket when I go to the movies.

–A. J. Fenner, age 18

Tip: Take extra money for food when you go to the movies.

–Ant Engeln, age 14

Thinking Activities

Heavy concentration requires lots of glucose (sugar). Be prepared—exams and long tournaments require many snacks and frequent tests. You can get low.

- Treat an intense intellectual activity just like you would an intense athletic one.
- Test before exams and other intellectual activities.

Spike's Chess Tournament

When I was in kindergarten, I decided I wanted to enter the school chess tournament. The only problem was that I didn't know how to play. I asked my parents to teach me, and they got out the checkerboard. I think my dad told me something about how chess was too complicated for a five-year-old. Now I'm pretty sure he just didn't know how to play.

I was enamored by all things medieval and was determined to enter the tournament (I thought, and still think, any game with knights and castles has to be cool), and I didn't want to lose. Finding no help from my parents, who thought it was too hard, no help from my sisters, who were more interested in watching Punky Brewster in those days, and no help from Bo, who was only three, after all, I turned to my only alternative—*World Book Encyclopedia.*

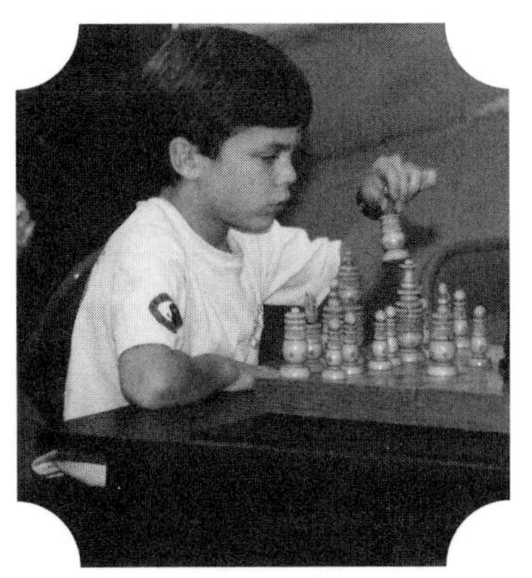

Spike Loy

Our encyclopedia had diagrams of how the pieces moved, pictures of famous chess players, and directions on how to play. I stayed up in my room reading one night, and challenged my dad to a game the next morning. I won. I think I had to show him the rules a few times during the game but a win is a win.

That day at school I announced to my teacher, who was also the principal and organizer of the school chess tournament, that I wanted to enter. He said anyone could enter but he warned me not to expect too much, since the sixth-graders usually won. I wasn't fazed. I stayed up that night reading all the articles in our *World Book* that were listed in the appendix as related topics to the *Chess* entry.

My parents decided I was serious about learning chess and brought out my Grandpa's ancient wooden board. It was awesome. The pieces were all handcrafted and painted. Sure it was a little dusty but like I said, no one in my house had played a game of chess in a long time. They also bought a book on chess for beginners. I stayed up late reading this book, and my parents stayed up late trying to figure out all the rules so they could help me with my new passion. After a week they had mastered the rules of the game, and I could beat both my mom and my dad even when they played on the same team. Actually, it was easier to beat them when they were on the same team because they would talk to each other about what they planned to do and give away any tiny bit of strategy their puny minds had to begin with. Suckers. It made them so mad to lose to little Spikey. I loved it, and before long my parents signed me up with a private chess teacher.

At my elementary school, there was a 4th, 5th, and 6th grade tournament. I won the 4th grade tournament (they wouldn't let me enter with the 6th graders . . . yet). The winners from each grade got to go to the district championship and compete against kids at other schools. Since I won the fourth grade level chess tournament at Summit Elementary School, my principal decided I would get to play against the kids who won at other schools at the big district tournament. I showed up with the fifth- and sixth-graders from my school and the principals from the other schools all kind of laughed at the little kindergartner. That was *me*, and it kinda ticked me off. I won my first game, and the kid I beat cried. I felt bad about that, but it felt good to see the other schools' principals quit laughing. I won the next two games and, after winning the third one in just under a minute, I was the Ojai Unified School District's Fourth Grade Chess Champion! I got my picture in the *Ojai Valley News* and everything.

In first, second, and third grades, I defended my title as the fourth-grade chess champion. I couldn't be beat! I was invincible! When I won at Summit in fourth grade, I was extra excited to go to the district tournament and finally be playing against kids who were actually my own age. I knew a lot of these guys from Little League or soccer and wanted to beat them at chess *real bad*. I won the first two games without a problem but I remember making some pretty dumb mistakes during my third game. My mom remembered that, too, and said she just thought I was tired and not paying much attention. I won that game but it was closer than it should have been. Then came my fifth championship game in five years, and this time I was actually a few months *older* than my opponent.

It should have been a cinch. I started with my normal opening and after a few minutes was down three pieces. I was *never* down three pieces. I started getting worried and playing sloppily. I knocked pieces off the table by accident, reaching out with shaky hands. I didn't know what was wrong, but I remember thinking that I was actually going to lose. I did, too. I lost to Jake. I knew Jake from soccer, and we had played chess on the bus to all-star games. I had never lost to him. But I lost that day.

When he checkmated me, he was thrilled. "I beat Spike!" he shouted and his principal gave him a big hug. I wanted to cry.

My mom thought I was just upset at losing, but when she tried to talk to me, and I wouldn't say anything back she got to thinking it might be a little something more. We tested. I was only 40! No wonder I wasn't talking. My blood sugar was super low. I could barely even stand, much less play a championship chess game against a good opponent like Jake. I ate while the trophies were being handed out, and once I felt better I congratulated Jake.

We realized that day just how important blood sugar can be for activities that exercise your brain. Your brain uses a lot of sugar, just like your muscles. It was exactly the same as when I did badly on a test in class because my sugar was low. There just wasn't enough sugar in my blood to think as hard as I needed to think to play a game like chess.

I went back in fifth grade with a full stomach, snacks between games, and Gatorade on the table beside the chessboard, and I won easily. In sixth grade, I had a few tough games but won. That year, Bo entered the fourth-grade tournament with snacks, granola bars, and Gatorade, and he beat every kid he played, too. That was the first year Summit school ever won the whole tournament. Bo and I each got trophies, and our school got one to keep in the display case in the office. It was pretty cool.

- Check your blood sugar and snack-up before chess tournaments, academic decathlons, exams, and important intellectual events like taking the SATs.
- Take a snack or Gatorade to exams and competitions.

Acting and Performing

Dancing

Mollie has been dancing for 11 years: jazz, hip-hop, ballet, tap, and lyrical. Her dance team has competed in Star Power (the biggest dance competition in the world) once or twice a year for the past 7 years, traveling to Orlando, Nashville, Fort Lauderdale, Houston, and Atlanta. Recently they were booked as the entertainment on a cruise ship to the Bahamas.

Mollie: I just went on the pump this year, and I like my pump a lot. Last year, dancing every day of the week on injections, it was hard for me to keep up. When dance class ran from 4:00 PM to 7:00 PM, I would have to stop and go eat, and I would miss something. With the pump, I can eat right before class or right after, and it won't mess up my schedule too much. Plus, my A1C level was creeping up a little bit, and now it is coming down. I just love being on the pump!

I wear my pump during practice when we are dancing or just doing routines, but when we start doing stunts, I disconnect so nobody will get tangled up in the tubing. (I wear the shortest tubing you can get, so I have less tubing to take care of.)

It's a little more complicated when we are competing. I might be wearing a full body costume with layers and layers of clothes. Plus, in competitions we dance 15 numbers in 2 hours, back to back to back. *I make it work by being very organized.* I check my blood sugar after every two or three dances. If I need carbs, I drink juice or eat a little snack. State law requires that I disconnect my pump during performances, so I disconnect right before I go on stage—and the minute I'm off the stage, I hook back up.

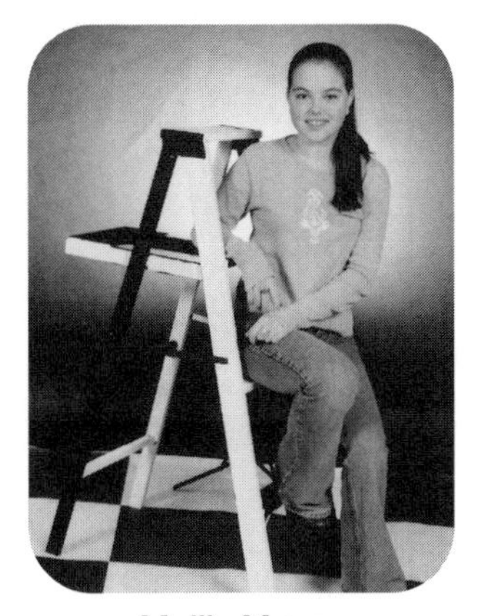

Mollie Meggs

When the dance team travels, I pack and then my mom double-checks. I have to make sure I take every costume, every prop, every little accessory, *and* all my diabetes supplies. My mom goes through everything to make sure it's in order. Sometimes she writes a list of what supplies we have and what we need to take along on the trip. *–Mollie Meggs, age 14*

Playing music

Brendan Black is a jazz musician. When we met Brendan at a teen retreat at UCLA, he shared his insights on playing the sax.

Spike and Bo: Performing and playing music is definitely a *physical activity*, it is *exciting*, and you can also have *performance anxiety*, three things that may lower blood sugars.

Before a performance I test and snack up as usual. I like to be at 160 when I step out on the stage or sit down for a gig. For a two- or three-hour performance I usually have something to drink, like Gatorade. Gatorade is good stuff. A bottle of Gatorade might last an hour. Then I test at intermission. Depending on the test results, I might have to take a couple units (or bolus) to cover the Gatorade, or if I'm low, I snack on something.

- Be aware of where your numbers are before you step onstage. You never know how performing is going to affect you.
- Have Gatorade close at hand.
- I've noticed that performing makes you thirsty so drink lots of water, too. *–Brendan Black, age 19*

When our friend Andy Savage, a water polo player and fellow surfer, isn't in the water, he plays bass guitar in a band, *Cavil at Rest*.

Andy: Our practice sessions (in my friend Ryan's garage) are energetic and usually last for about two hours. I test before and after each session—I have pretty good control on the pump testing before and after each session. On stage we play Rock n' Roll with heart. I guess you could say the way we perform is definitely exercise. I always keep a can of real soda close by just in case I get that feeling. If I feel kind of shaky, or maybe a little confused, or if everything gets blurry, I know I'm low, and I drink some soda. I also keep a backpack just offstage filled with extra food, granola bars, and juice.

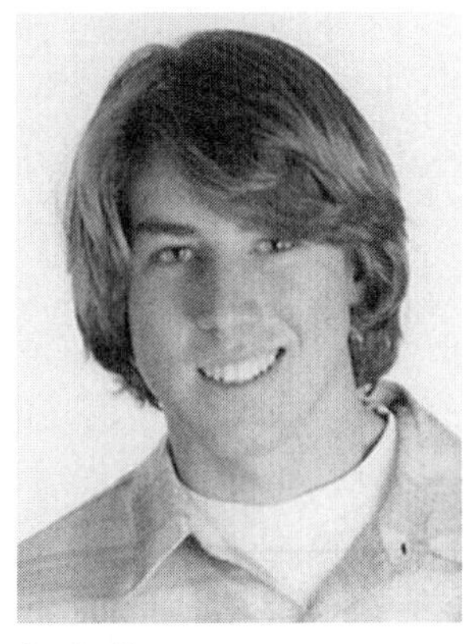

Andy Savage

- Keep a sugary drink within reach when you're onstage.

–Andy Savage, age 15

Tip: Before acting (or any activity where you are on the stage) eat some carbohydrates, because when you get nervous, you can get low. *–Vanessa Flores, age 16*

Tip: When you are acting, always have a sugary drink or candy with you. *–Shalee Penner, age 14*

High School and the Teen Years

Dealing with diabetes at high school is just like dealing with it in elementary and middle school. You still need to let all of your teachers know about it, and you still need to be prepared and have lots of food around. Since you're older, and hopefully smarter (neither of us can vouch for the other on this one) and have more freedom, diabetes can be easier to manage. You have more options and can handle more things on your own if you want to.

- Request a locker. Even if your school doesn't have a locker for everyone, if you tell them you need one to keep your food in for diabetes, they'll give you one. It's nice to be able to put your books away while all your friends lug them around all day, too!

- If you drive yourself to school, keep a cooler in your car. If you hitch a ride with a friend, keep a cooler in their car and ask them for a spare key.
- Tell each of your new teachers that you have diabetes and give them a copy of *Symptoms* (page 250). Tell them when you are having lows.

Spike: Of course, just because you are older and can take care of more stuff on your own doesn't mean you *have* to, or even that you should. Even when I was 16, my mom still met with my teachers before the school year started and told them about lows and highs and what to do. It was nice not having to deal with that stuff until I was ready (my junior year). Bo handled a lot more on his own. I think it was because I (actually, Mom) had already warmed the teachers up, but Bo insists he is just more mature than I am.

Anyway, it is nice to be a kid as long as you can, and to let your parents help when they can. I remember getting annoyed by my mom when I was 17, and she would still come to my soccer games and wait on the sidelines with Gatorade. I remember when I was 18, and she would insist that my friend, Andrew, stick a granola bar in his pocket and not eat it "or else" before we would go out to a party. Maybe I got annoyed, but it sure was nice to have someone else helping me out. Thanks, Mom!

- Let your parents take care of as much as they want to and help you out for as long as they can. Someday you'll be on your own and, trust me, you will wish they were still helping you remember your kit and cooler, or making you scrambled eggs and bacon, so you could have a healthy, high protein breakfast.

- If your friends know what's going on, they will be eager to help.
- Let your friends be part of your team by having them guess your sugar and figure out whether you need calories or insulin.

Tip: Make sure all your teachers are educated about diabetes, especially coaches. *–Anna Gleason, age 15*

Tip: When people don't know anything about diabetes, tell them about it. *–Alexie Milton, age 14*

Tip: Make sure your teachers know you have diabetes and what your low blood sugar symptoms are. If you're low, don't wait! Leave class if you have to and test or eat. *–Anita Kaura, age 17*

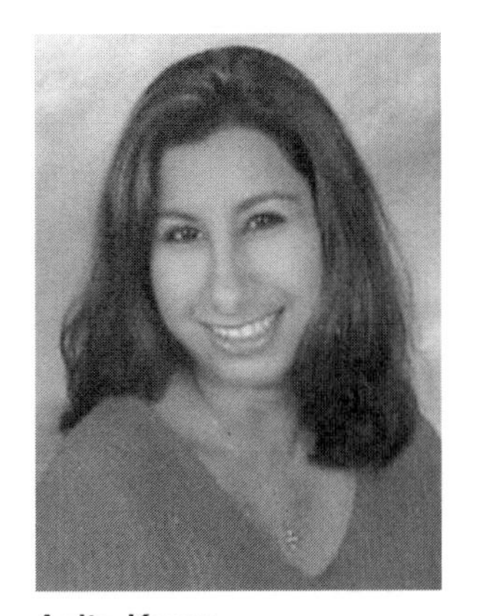

Anita Kaura

Tip: I use a beeper case that clips onto my waistband for my emergency supplies. I keep my glucose and medical ID in it, so I don't lose them. The case is really good for PE, since my PE clothes don't have any pockets. *–Joe DeMario, age 13*

Tip: When I get low, I just take out a glucose tablet and eat it without disturbing the class. *–Joe DeMario, age 13*

Tip: Carry a fun-size candy in your purse. *–Valerie Kintz, age 15*

Bullies

Spike: There was a bully in my middle school. If you wore glasses, he made fun of you for that. If you were short (and I was), he made fun of you for that. If you were tall, yup, you got made fun of. Well, I was short and had diabetes, so I used to get it from him quite a bit. He thought he was real tough and used to fight a lot, too, so punching him in the nose was basically out of the question. I had to outsmart him.

There are lots of different ways of dealing with kids who make fun of you for having diabetes, but my favorite is to scare them half to death. If someone is making fun of you and you just ignore them, sometimes that is enough to get them to stop. But sometimes it might not be enough. When I was growing up, there were a few times when people continued pestering me even after I ignored everything they said.

Confront them

One day I was testing my blood sugar at lunch in the cafeteria. This guy comes up and says something like "Hey, Shorty, your diabetes contagious?" I looked up at him and just said, "Yes, yes it is," and then I coughed on him. All of my friends who were sitting and eating at my table knew it wasn't contagious—but he didn't! He never bugged me again.

Educate them

Being open and honest about your diabetes is the best way to avoid having to confront bullies. The more people who understand that I can do anything, the fewer people there are out there who are ignorant enough to make fun of me. People who understand that my life is, at times, a little bit harder than theirs usually want to help instead of hurt.

Ask for help

If you try to educate a bully and it doesn't work, and you don't want to have a big confrontation, you can always tell a teacher or the principal. Usually they will talk to the kid in question and straighten him or her right up. Also, don't be afraid to let your parents call the school or even the other kid's parents. There is no reason you should have to deal with some mean-spirited brat all on your own. (Lastly, if the kid's parents aren't cooperative, or the school isn't cooperative, your parents could threaten to sue them. That might work.)

- Tell a teacher or administrator if someone is really bothering you.
- Let your parents know when someone is being mean to you. They can often handle the situation and leave you free to be a kid.

Tip: Some people act weirded out the first time they see my pump. I take a minute and just tell them the truth, that this is like my pancreas, but it's on the outside. With just this little bit of knowledge, they become part of my team. *–Jessica Stogsdill, age 18*

Spike: Bo and I always call our kits our "purses." One of our friends is bound to make the joke sooner or later, and if we start the joke, it kind of steals their thunder.

Cars and Driving

Bo: At the PADRE Teen Retreat we met wild and crazy Dr. Tim Flannery. In between skits, practical jokes, and water polo lessons, he gave us a great tip about driving: "You don't drive a car without your driver's license, right? Well, if you have diabetes, you don't drive a car without your medical ID. Simple as that."

- Don't go on a car ride without a cooler—if you forget it, go back and get it.
- When you get picked up by a neighbor, or go off in a friend's car, or otherwise change cars, take your cooler with you.
- Keep a bottle of Gatorade on the front seat beside you. If you get low and are stuck in traffic, you can reach for your Gatorade.
- If you even think you may be low, pull over to the side of the road, test and snack-up. Wait until your blood sugar is back to normal before driving.
- Have a card in your wallet stating you have diabetes and that if you seem disoriented, you need sugar. That way if you are in low blood sugar trouble and an officer stops you, he/she can offer you some calories.

Tip: Toss a tube of Cake Mate frosting in the glove compartment of all the cars you ride in. *–Matt Egizi, age 9*

Tip: Keep candy in the car, so if you get low, you know where to find some fast-acting sugar.
–Kelly Hrubeniuk, age 10

Tip: Keep candy and granola bars in your car.
–Anna Gleason, age 15

Tip: Test before driving, *before* you get into the car. The chances of forgetting to test are much higher if you wait until you are behind the wheel.
–Brendan Black, age 19

Dating

Spike: Throughout high school all of my girlfriends (not that there were that many of them) knew I had diabetes long before we ever got romantic. They were friends of mine, and everyone at my school knew my brother and I had diabetes. It was never a big deal at all. They would put granola bars in their purses and never got upset if I had to swing by McDonald's on the way to a movie to keep from getting low. When I went away to college, however, my girlfriend Vanessa didn't know I had diabetes until our first date.

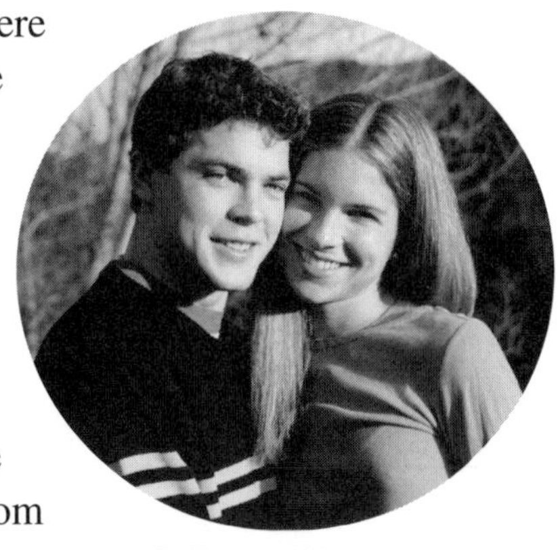

Spike and Vanessa

I had talked to this girl at a few parties and finally got the nerve to ask her out on an official date. She said yes (thank heavens), and I decided to take her to a real nice restaurant in downtown Palo Alto. I showed up at her door promptly at 7:30. Of course she wasn't ready, and I spent the first of many hundreds of hours waiting for Vanessa to get ready. (It was well worth the wait—she looked stunning.) We got to the restaurant a bit late, but luckily, they hadn't given away our table yet.

Vanessa didn't say anything about the kit I brought in to the restaurant, and I didn't mention anything to her until I tested my blood.

"Oh, by the way, I have diabetes. Right now I am just checking my blood to see how much insulin I am going to need to shoot up."

"Oh, cool. I was wondering why you had a purse." (Guys, someone is bound to call your kit a "purse" someday. Around smart-alecky friends who consider themselves witty and clever, I always call my kit my purse. It beats them to the punch and leaves them with nothing to say.)

Back to the date—my sugar was a tiny bit low. (I think it must have been nerves, but I didn't tell Vanessa that. I was still trying to act cool and in control of myself and our relationship . . . what a joke.) So I ate a generous helping of bread and waited until our meals arrived to shoot up. I explained to Vanessa a bit about highs and lows and let her watch me inject when the food got there. Other than the 60 seconds it took me to test, the two minutes we talked about what a blood sugar was and the 10 seconds it took me to inject, diabetes never came up for the rest of the night. To be honest with you, I think she forgot all about it until we got up to leave, and I almost forgot my purse. (Nerves, I tell you.)

Tip: Don't worry about telling a date you have diabetes. If they see that you are responsible and in charge, they'll like you even more. *–Jenna Rohm, age 16*

Tip: I tell my dates up front that I have diabetes and what can happen if I get low, and I suggest that they give me some orange juice or apple juice if they think I'm low. *–Diana Cibrian, age 16*

Tip: As far as dating goes, don't worry about it! I've had diabetes for seven years and I've realized that being upfront about diabetes is always the best. Just tell your date you are a diabetic and they should be cool with it. If they're not, you probably don't want to date them anyway. *–Brooks Kincaid, age 21*

Jennifer: For some odd reason, I worried about what guys would think about a girl who had diabetes. My thinking was crazy. Having diabetes hasn't interfered with dating at all. Just like with friends, take a little time, and educate your dates.

My first boyfriend didn't have a clue when he saw me take a shot before dinner. I forgot that lots of people don't know anything about diabetes. So I explained to him that I inject insulin, that when I get low, I need to drink some juice and relax, then

I'd be myself again. It didn't faze him—he was really understanding, and always a great help when I needed it.

- When you spend a lot of time with someone, help them to understand diabetes. *People who care about you want to help.* Be patient and don't expect them to know everything right away. *–Jennifer Ogden, age 19*

Tip: Carry candy in your purse when you go on a date. *–Diana Cibrian, age 16*

Tip: When I went to prom, I was on injections. I didn't want to carry anything but I wanted to have sugar with me, so I put my glucose tablets in my stocking—and left my *little* diabetes kit in the car. I ate some long-lasting protein and fat before prom. They served a sit-down dinner, and I was fine. Plus, I had my kit and a snack waiting for me in the car. *–Jessica Stogsdill, age 18*

Tip: Getting low when you are on a date can be a little bit of a problem, especially when you have good control. All those hormones rushing around can cause your sugar to crash. Just the anticipation of kissing can cause low blood sugars. In anticipation of an exciting date, you can lower your insulin or keep a snack around. I like Gatorade. *–Mary Costello, age 21*

Tip: If kissing or making out is spontaneous, the excitement can *really* make you low, so pause and drink some Gatorade. *–Mary Costello, age 21*

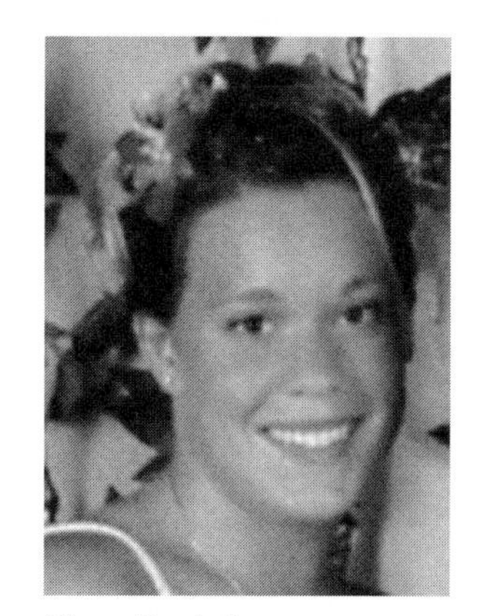

Mary Costello

Tip: When you have good control, you've got less leeway before you are low. Make carrying sugar and Gatorade part of your dating routine. *–Mary Costello, age 21*

Tip: If you know you are going to be intimate, say in an hour, you can reduce your basal if you're on the pump. If you are on injections, you may need a snack.
–Mary Costello, age 21

Tip: Don't worry if you're on a pump, it's just like a piece of clothing. If you're ever in a situation where you need to remove it, just disconnect—it's like taking off a sweater.
–Mary Costello, age 21

Everything We Know about Going Off to College

Applying to different schools, visiting campuses, and getting ready to move out of the house for the first time is a little hectic and a lot of fun. It's also a lot of work. Having diabetes meant we had to work just a little harder and be a little bit more organized than our friends. With organization, you can do anything you want to. Here is a list of important tips to help make your transition from home to college as smooth as possible:

- Go ahead and mark the "handicapped" or "chronically ill" box on your applications. This will let the school know that you have a condition that may require special attention, and it will make life easier once you start school. It won't hurt your admissions status either.
- Register at the disabilities office.

We don't for a second consider diabetes to be a handicap. It hasn't kept us from surfing, going on 100-mile bike rides, traveling in third-world countries, playing all-star sports, or anything else; but registering will ensure you get the support you need, if and when you need it. It will also help you get preferred housing.

- Get housing with an open kitchen or that is near 24-hour food.

Your daily routine will change when you go off to school. College students stay up a lot later just about every night (sometimes even to study), and when you are up late, you need to eat something late at night, too. It's nice to be able to eat some prepared food and not have to settle for something out of a box every night.

- Put a small refrigerator in your room.

This is something we really think is important. We both have refrigerators in our rooms. We use them to keep our insulin, ice packs, and glucagon kits cool, and we store our favorite foods in them to boot. String cheese for snacking and a small carton of orange juice for low blood sugars. We've just learned that glucagon doesn't have to be refrigerated any longer, so you can keep it in your diabetes drawer or cooler.

- Get a meal plan that has no absolute limit.

Sometimes an unlimited meal plan can cost a little extra, but assuring easy access to food every day is important. Plus, you will probably be able to sell some of your extra points to your less-prepared friends.

- Don't be afraid to use special resources that your new school may offer you.

Spike: At Stanford, as a registered diabetic, I could have a note-taker, hired by the school, take notes for me in any class I missed due to low blood sugars or late nights dealing with ketones. I never needed to use this service, but it was nice to know it was there. I did, however, get to make up a test I missed because I had stayed up the whole night before handling some real low sugars. I just let my professor know via e-mail that I wasn't going to be able to make it, and since he knew I had diabetes he rescheduled it for the next day.

- We can't stress too much how important it is to let everyone around you know that you have diabetes.

My new roommate knew I had diabetes before he knew my name. That's because he saw the large Sparklett's water bottle full of used syringes I kept beneath my bed. The rest of my dorm mates found out at our first dinner, when I pricked my finger and shot up. To be honest, it was a pretty good way to meet people. Most everyone knows someone who has diabetes, and kids at colleges tend to want to know more about it. I always tell everyone the basics and a little bit about what the symptoms of lows are and what they should do if they think I am low.

We recommend going a bit further with the staff of your dorm and your close friends who will be around all the time:

- Hand out a list of symptoms of low blood sugars to your RAs and other staff members. List your symptoms: dizziness, irritability, faintness, and absentmindedness (*Symptoms*, page 250).
- Give your dorm staff a list of things to do if they think you are low. Things like getting you some sugar, real Coke or juice, putting frosting on your gums if you can't or won't eat, and calling 911 if anything major should ever come up.

Spike: I feel it is important to let the staff know that, although I rarely need help with low blood sugars, it is sure nice knowing that there are a few other people around who know what is going on and who are on my team.

- Print out a list detailing how to use a glucagon kit (page 253).

Bo: I still have my list inside my closet, and everyone I live with knows where it is. It is also a good idea to set up your dorm room, so you can always get to your needles and meter easily. Here is how Spike and I set our rooms up:

- Buy a set of plastic drawers and designate one or two of them as your Diabetes Drawer.
- Keep your needles, lancets, strips, and meter in your Diabetes Drawer as well as granola bars, a box of crackers, a box of cookies, and a Gatorade for lows.
- Get a big Sharps container or water bottle to store your needles.

It's convenient to have a place right next to your fridge where you can toss your used needles after you inject. It will also amaze your friends to see how many syringes you go through in a semester.

- Make sure you tell your friends that some of your food is *totally off limits*.

Trust me, you will have to tell some of them several dozen times before they quit asking for granola bars. I decided it was easier to go ahead and buy an extra box of crackers that I could share now and then and still keep plenty stashed for late night lows.

As you go through college, you'll figure out what works best for you, and before long you'll have your routine down and diabetes won't get in your way one bit. As we always say, you can do anything with diabetes, you just have to be a little bit smarter and more prepared than your friends.

Things to do before going to college

- Visit the college campus.
- Visit the Students with Disabilities Office. Ask for their advice.
- Mark "Disabled Student" on your college application.
- Enroll in the college's student health insurance program even if you already have good insurance.
- When filling out housing request forms, make sure you mark special housing needs. Ask for housing on campus and near a food supply. Send forms in on time!
- Start Hepatitis B series of inoculations 6 months before school starts.
- Some schools recommend a meningitis vaccination.
- Get a flu shot before leaving for college or while on campus.

Right before leaving for college, visit the campus again

- Locate places to eat, cafeterias, coffee shops, food venues open all night.
- Locate the student health center.
- Locate the nearest emergency room to your dorm.
- Make an appointment with a doctor at the student health service center before school starts or during the first week of school. Ask your regular doctor to have your diabetes-related records sent to him/her.
- Have all diabetes-related prescriptions sent to the school pharmacy before school starts. Phone to make sure your prescriptions are in place.

Supplies to take to college:

A room refrigerator stocked with:

- Insulin
- Glucagon (this is essential)
- Cottage cheese, whole milk, string cheese
- A typed list of emergency phone numbers (tape it to the phone), including:
  - Parents
  - Doctor
  - Endocrinologist
  - School clinic
  - Adult brothers and sisters
- Glucagon instruction sheet (another essential)
- Symptoms instruction sheet
- Insulin kit
- Ketone test strips
- Medical I.D.
- Blue Ice cold packs—two
- Cooler—packed for car trips
- A huge box of snacks, including:
  - Jerky
  - Crackers
  - Cookies
  - Cup-O-Noodles
  - Nuts
  - Frosting, candy, glucose tablets
- A second set of:
  - Insulin
  - Syringes
  - Meter batteries
  - Blood testing strips or discs
  - Chemstrips

➠ **Note:** *Real Life Parenting of Kids with Diabetes* devotes an entire chapter to going off to college, including the above lists and tips for kids and parents!

College is a big change for kids who may have grown up with their parents hounding them to take care of themselves. In college it is all your responsibility. When kids get here, they may not always check their blood as often as they should. They start to wake up at two in the afternoon, which will surely screw up any kid's insulin schedule; hey, it happened to me when I got here. The most important thing is to be responsible for your own health.

- Carry your insulin, glucose checker, etc. with you. If you feel uncomfortable carrying something around that people might think is a purse, then put it in your backpack, and take that with you.
- Wake up at a decent hour to take your insulin and eat, even if you just go back to sleep and miss your class.

–Rory Tarbox, age 19

Bryan Kam, 17, is attending Princeton. Yeah, we know, he's 17 years old, and he's at an Ivy League school. We figured a kid this smart should have some helpful tips for other kids with diabetes going off to school. He sent us the following e-mail:

Spike and Bo,

The hardest part of adjusting to college life, for me, was the fact that my schedule changed. During high school, every day is pretty much the same, and during the summer, I worked a pretty regular schedule. So having classes at different hours, waking up at varying times, napping because I was writing a paper the night before, and skipping meals—all of these things made it tough to remember to test during the first days of college. I have to force myself to test at meals, rather than just hitting the buttons on my pump, in order to stay in good control.

Be careful with your insulin during the first month. I found myself walking much more than I previously had, and I was not used to the effect all that exercise had on my blood sugar. Those far-away classes can really put a dent in your blood sugar.

I also learned to buy candy that you don't like enough to devour while your blood sugar is normal, so you could keep it in your room. If I go low in the wee hours of the morning (12–4 AM), there are few places open to get food. It is much easier to have glucose on hand. The problem is if I keep food that I enjoy, I may eat it before I actually go low. I find that Necco Wafers work well—even if I start eating them, I usually get sick of them before I've exhausted a pack.

Most importantly, you need to just pay attention. On my campus, with so many activities, so much work, and so many great people to chill with, time doesn't just fly, it reaches about mach 4. Since I am on a pump, I have to be very careful to remember to change my site frequently. Even when I am cautious, I find myself asking, "Has it really been three days?" It seems like less than an hour.

–Bryan Kam, age 17

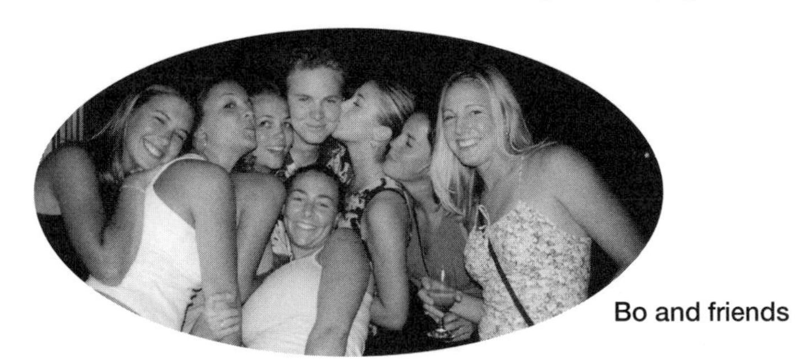

Bo and friends

Extracurricular activities

Drinking

Spike: Drinking a little bit of alcohol is one of those things that with diabetes, you really shouldn't do, but you might try anyway. There is a lot of sugar in beer, wine, and alcohol that you just don't need, and alcohol affects your body in all sorts of weird ways. If you have a beer from time to time, only drink in moderation and drink a lot more responsibly than your friends.

I always snack while I am drinking. This seems counter-intuitive, since I am eating more *while* I guzzle a sugar-filled drink, but it is very important. Your liver has two important jobs that are relevant here. First, it releases sugar into your blood when you aren't eating, like at night when you are asleep. Second, it acts as a filter and cleans all of the poisons (in this case, alcohol) out of your system. The problem is that while it is hard at work as a filter, it quits releasing sugar into your blood. So, although your blood sugar may skyrocket while you are drinking, it will come down and your liver will be too busy filtering alcohol and won't release any sugar into your system while you sleep, and you can crash big time.

- Always eat while you are drinking alcohol. Always!
- Alcohol can cause lower blood sugar 8 hours after your last drink. Factor in physical activity too, like dancing all night—because warm muscles absorb sugar too.

You may also want to lower your nighttime insulin dose a bit (especially if you use NPH) if you are going to drink. This will help make sure you don't crash in the middle of the night and that you wake up the next morning. Of course, with all the sugar in the alcohol, the extra food you are snacking on, and less insulin, there is a good chance you will be high for most of the night and that's just not healthy.

- Always, always eat a bedtime snack after drinking and check your blood sugar (about 10 grams of carb per beer). This will help keep your sugars from dropping in the early hours of the morning while your liver is busy detoxifying your system.

The key with drinking is to only do it in moderation. If you only drink a beer or two, you won't have to worry about your liver quitting on you, and you can treat the carbs like you would any food.

- If you are going to drink, drink light beer. It has fewer carbs.

If you don't overdo it and you only drink once in a while, you should be fine. If you drink too much *even once,* you could run into serious trouble. Tell all of your friends to watch out for you and to make sure you eat. Tell them how to use glucagon and to call 911 if you ever pass out. If you throw up, follow the same guidelines you do when you throw up because you are sick. Let someone know right away if you throw up once, and if it happens twice, call for help.

Of course, all of these problems can be avoided if you don't drink. Plus, if you stay sober, you can take pictures of all your friends making fools of themselves and blackmail them later.

Tip: When I drink just one beer, I don't notice any change in my numbers. *–Mary Costello, age 21*

Tip: Tell your friends to call 911 if you ever pass out, even if they think it's alcohol related. It's possible your diabetes needs help. *–Mary Costello, age 21*

Tip: Make sure you have your glucometer. When you drink, you need to test often to make sure your blood sugar is not going too high or too low. Dancing, walking around, or going to sleep late, combined with alcohol, can all make your blood sugar go down, despite all of the carbohydrates in booze. Taking a test kit around with you to a party can be annoying, but it is essential. I usually just put my kit in my pocket until I get to where I am going. Then I put my kit somewhere I know I'll be able to find it later. *–Brooks Kincaid, age 21*

Tip: Don't drink beyond your limit. Especially in high school and college, people have a tendency to drink until they're wasted, and end up throwing up. For diabetics, this is a bad scenario. Drinking to that stage can really mess up your blood sugar. If you do screw up and drink to that point, it's not the end of the world but you have to be extra careful. After vomiting you'll need to test, then eat and drink sugary drinks. Make sure the people you are with know you have diabetes and that you need to eat. And make sure to TEST. *–Brooks Kincaid, age 21*

Tip: If you are new to the pump, do not add in the carbohydrate from an alcoholic beverage when calculating your insulin bolus. Alcohol typically causes hypoglycemia. Eat when you drink alcohol and test often, every 30 to 60 minutes. *–Mary Costello, age 21*

Tip: Make sure you have access to food. Your blood sugar is harder to gauge when you drink. If it goes low (or even if you think it might), you want to be able to have a snack before going to bed. *–Brooks Kincaid, age 21*

Tip: As far as drinking goes, stay away from mixed drinks as much as possible. You never know what is in them, and they're often very sugary. *–Brooks Kincaid, age 21*

Tip: If you don't want to drink, let your friends know, and it shouldn't be a big deal. *–Rory Tarbox, age 19*

Bo and I had a deal with our parents. They didn't want us going out and doing anything stupid, but the deal was this: If we ever got into trouble, we could call, or our friends could call, and they would come help out—no questions asked. Parents would rather you do the right thing and call them than be afraid to call and get into really bad trouble. Make a deal with your parents, and call them if you drink too much.

Smoking

Spike: We all know that smoking is bad for you. It's bad for everybody. It's addictive and screws up your body. And girls, no one will ever want to kiss you when your breath smells like smoke. Trust me on this one.

Smoking cigarettes is even worse for you when you have diabetes. Nicotine causes problems with the tiny blood vessels in your arms and legs, and diabetes does that too (if you have lots of really high blood sugars for long periods of time). One of the worst things someone with diabetes can do is take up smoking. Do not smoke!

That said, I will admit that I have tried cigarettes and cigars, and even chewing tobacco. Don't ask me why I ever tried chewing tobacco. I think I had some in my mouth for all of 30 seconds before I turned green and had to excuse myself to the bathroom. I won't be trying that again. Cigarettes I *hate*. I can count on one hand how many times I have tried cigarettes. You're better off chewing dirt than smoking cigarettes as far as I am concerned.

Cigars I treat kind of like birthday cake. When I go to a birthday party, I let myself bend my rules a little bit. I don't eat a great big piece of cake, but I'll go ahead and have a real small one. Plus I will do my best not to eat all the icing. Similarly, once in a very rare while, I have half of a cigar. For instance, I smoked a cigar after I graduated from college in March (I smoked the second half of it four months later on the 4th of July). Again, using tobacco is one of the worst things you can do to yourself as a diabetic. Even *trying* cigarettes can be dangerous if you get addicted. If you feel that you are the kind of person who does get addicted to things, you can skip this experience. Your best bet is to just leave tobacco to kids who have money to waste and not a whole lot of brains to waste it with.

Marijuana

It's illegal, and smoking pot also has serious consequences for your diabetes. There is always the chance that you would be so out of it after smoking that you wouldn't be able to take care of yourself. If you miss a shot, your sugars would end up super high, and you might get ketones. That can quickly get dangerous. If you miss a snack, and have insulin in your system, you could be in even more serious trouble. Even if you aren't totally out of it, you might get the munchies and drive your sugar up, and that's just not healthy.

Even though marijuana is illegal, it's around at parties. Just because other people don't pass out when they are high doesn't mean it would affect you the same. If you do try it, only try a little, and check your blood sugar afterwards. Lower your insulin dosage beforehand in case you get really messed up, and make sure to snack so you don't bottom out. Let the friends who are with you know about glucagon and tell them to call 911 if they can't wake you up. It is always better to prepare for the worst. Are they responsible enough to take care of you?

- Go ahead and call your parents if you mess up or get into a situation you don't know how to handle.

Friends

Tell your friends about diabetes, and let them be on your team. When friends know about low blood sugars, they will want to help. Our friends used to be curious about blood tests, so we let them check their blood sugar (with a new lancet for each one of course). Once you start talking about diabetes, kids ask all kinds of questions. Don't be offended if a kid asks if he can get diabetes from you. Just tell them no, diabetes is not contagious.

Tip: Tell your friends about diabetes, so they can help you out. *–Catilini Ceballos, age 11*

Tip: Make sure friends, acquaintances, teachers, and people you work with are aware of your diabetes.

–Katherine Gresch, age 16

Tip: Explain to your friends or roommates that sometimes high or low blood sugars can make you feel out-of-sorts, and that you may need 10–20 minutes or so to get your rosy disposition back. I get really crabby at times (and not just during low blood sugars).

–Jennifer Ogden, age 19

Tip: Get family and friends involved and excited about your diabetes and diabetes management. *–Derrick Crowe, age 8*

Tip: Find a friend with diabetes. They always understand what you're going through. *–Jenna Rohm, age 16*

Tip: Make and keep friends who have diabetes as you do. They offer priceless friendship and support.

–A.J. Fenner, age 18

Tip: I tell the friends I hang out with to give me sugar if I get shaky or act really low. My friends know I always carry glucose tabs in my backpack. *–Laura Reichstadt, age 14*

Tip: Ask your friends if it's all right to do blood tests and shots in front of them. They will be interested.

–Dani Nelson, age 14

Tip: Reach out and help someone else. It puts it all in perspective. *–Kirk Barnette, age 21*

Tip: My brother Brian carries a snack wherever we go. Then if I get low, he can give it to me. My 5 brothers and sisters look out for me! *–Matt Egizi, age 9*

Tip: DJ, my best friend, comes into the office with me to check my sugar. One time my sugar was at 32. DJ stayed while I ate three glucose tablets. Then we went to the cafeteria and had lunch. Let your friends help.

–Cory Graham, age 12

Tip: Go ahead and ask your friends to carry a granola bar on hikes, outings, skiing, etc. Then if they notice that you are low, they can hand you something to eat.

–Evan McMillian, age 10

Share all you know about diabetes with your friends and other kids at school. More often than not they will be fascinated with your blood sugar tests, insulin, and carb balancing.

- Let other kids watch you test and get involved in helping figure out what you need. Insulin dosages and carbohydrates are things they can learn about too.
- Kids ask all kinds of questions. Don't be offended if kids ask you about AIDS. Be prepared with an answer. You know you don't have AIDS, so they can't get it from you. But remind them not to handle old syringes that they might find in the trash.
- Give a copy of *Symptoms* (page 250) to all your friends, teachers, coaches, and friends' parents. That way they can be part of your team and help.
- Let your friends give you a shot if they want to try it. Sometimes it's nice getting one in the arm for a change.

Helping Other Kids

You know, all kids with diabetes can reach out and help other kids. You can start out by sharing some of your know-how with one other kid, or you can go to a Kids With Diabetes convention and meet other kids and share ideas. You can advocate on the golf course, be on TV, or even go to Washington, D.C., for the ADA Call to Congress. Here is some sage advice on how to help other kids from our awesome friend, Jessica Stogsdill:

- When you share tips and techniques with others, you always end up learning.
- If you know someone who was just diagnosed—type 1 or type 2, it doesn't matter—or if you know someone who is having trouble managing diabetes, talk to him or her. Better yet, write down some of the things you do with your diabetes. Chances are if it works for you, it will work for other kids, too.
- The best way to learn is to teach someone else.

–Jessica Stogsdill, age 19

Tip: When I talk to other kids with diabetes, it gives me a sense of comfort to know that someone else out there shares the same experiences and can actually find words to describe those darn episodes of high and low blood sugar. *–Rahwa, age 20*

Tip: I like attending diabetes conventions because I like to see all the cool new stuff. It's fun to get all the free stuff too. *–Samantha McGuigan, age 8*

Tip: One good thing about coming to the Kids With Diabetes Convention is I got to learn all about the pump.

–Megan Kaniasty, age 11

Bo and the congressman

I had an experience the other day that showed people take notice when you advocate for kids. My friend Sean and I were out on the golf course walking across the green. I was carrying the only three golf clubs I own (a hand-me-down putter, a 9-iron, and an old wood driver) when Sean said, "Hey, there's Congressman Gallegly. I hope he comes over and talks to me."

You would expect the congressman to know Sean because he's the best high school golfer in the county and had been in all the newspapers for breaking all kinds of records. Congressman Elton Gallegly did notice us and began walking over. Sean, getting ready to make a putt, was all smiles, when the congressman walked up and said, "Hi Bo! How's your game?"

"It's going fine, Congressman, how 'bout yours?" We talked a bit about a diabetes-related meeting we'd had together, and he invited me to join him for a round of golf.

When he walked away, Sean said to me, "How's your game? How's *your* game? Are you kidding! This is only the second time you've ever played golf in your life!"

Be an advocate

Chris and Cory Graham, two amazing kids from North Carolina, introduced us to their friend Hannah Smith, from Oregon. When Hannah heard there was going to be a book filled with tips for kids, she jumped right in.

> Dear Bo and Spike,
>
> Hi, my name is Hannah Smith, and I'm 11 years old and have had diabetes for 3 1/2 years. I heard you were writing a new book on diabetes and looking for input from kids, and I would be happy to help.
>
> When I was a Children's Congress 2001 delegate, Chris and Cory and I spent many hours chatting online before the actual event. You see, the Graham family is originally from Oregon. We are all about the same age, so we have a lot in common. Plus, Chris and Cory were very helpful to me with advice when I went on the pump in March of 2001.
>
> When I was on our local TV station recently, a reporter asked me how having diabetes has changed my life. I thought

for a second and then said, "Having diabetes hasn't changed my life really, I just have to prick my finger."

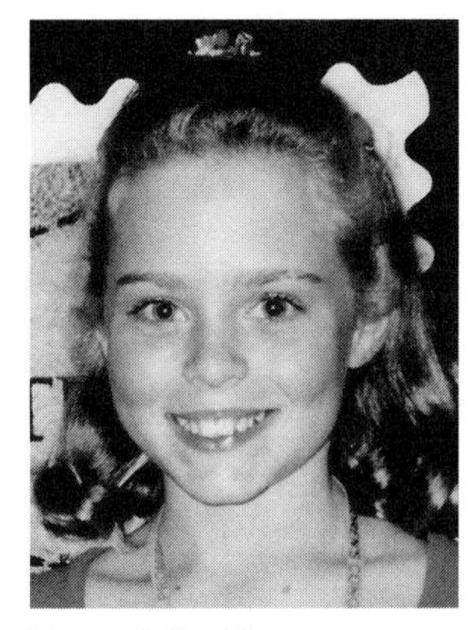

Hannah Smith

- The Children's Congress experience taught me that I am not too young to advocate for myself and other kids with diabetes.
  –Hannah Smith, age 11

Tip: Be an advocate. Talk to your congressman. They really listen to kids. (Don't be scared, the congressmen were pretty nervous too. They seemed more nervous than we were!) *–Chris & Cory Graham, ages 11 and 12*

Tip: When I met my congressman, my whole family came with me, and they got to meet him too. Advocating can be a family affair. *–Matt DiPaolo, age 10*

Tip: By raising money for the diabetes walk and getting a lot of awards for it, I have turned having diabetes into something positive. *–Danny Weiss, age 14*

Sharing

Bo: There is only a small chance that if one sibling has diabetes a brother or sister will also get it (our doc says 3–5%). Spike and I have diabetes but neither of our sisters, Mary nor Jenny, has it. Brothers Chris and Cory Graham, who both have diabetes, e-mailed us about having a sibling to look out for you.

Cory: When your brother has diabetes, there are two of you managing your stuff. It's a good support system. I try things first for Chris, because Chris is my younger brother, and I help him with his lows. When Chris was 6, he went to his first day camp, Camp KUDOS, in Charlotte, NC. He started to talk about how much fun he had. When he was done, I said, "I wish I had diabetes."

Well guess what? I got it. Chris had diabetes for 3 years before me, which was nice because we all knew what to do when I was diagnosed. And now I have Celiac. I wonder if Chris will get Celiac? It seems like we're always doing the same things. Later, Cory

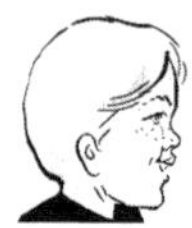

Cory has to avoid wheat and flour, things with gluten. He manages like a champ, and at 12 is already smarter than Spike.

Tip: I also have celiac. My mom and I go to a store that imports English food, and they have a lot of foods that are actually labeled as Gluten Free (unlike most American foods/snacks). *–Sophie Sheridan, age 9*

Chris: One time at school, Cory was low, and there were no sugars around, so I went right into the teachers' lounge and got some fast sugar food for Cory.

Cory: Another time Chris had a seizure. Mom and Dad gave him a glucagon shot while I called 911. He was fine. My brother and I help each other out a lot. It works both ways. If he had to, he could give someone a glucagon shot. So could I. Hope this helps your book.

Bo: Cory, I know exactly how you feel. Spike had diabetes for a full year before I was diagnosed, and he got a lot more attention than I did. I remember not only wishing I'd get it, but basically expecting that I would, because I did everything he did. It's kind of nice to have brothers to blaze the trail for us.

Thanks for the tips.

Your friend, Bo

Chris and Cory: We love the pump. There is less interference in your life—you can even sleep in. You can carry it in your pocket. You don't have to carry insulin and syringes everywhere you go. We think the pump is good for teenagers, because without the pump they need so many shots every day. The pump just gives you more freedom.

- It's nice to have pockets for your pump in the shorts you sleep in.
- Always carry some syringes even though you have a pump—just in case.
- Change your infusion site every three days. (A reminder that it's time to change your site is when your reservoir is getting low.)

–Chris and Cory Graham, ages 11 and 12

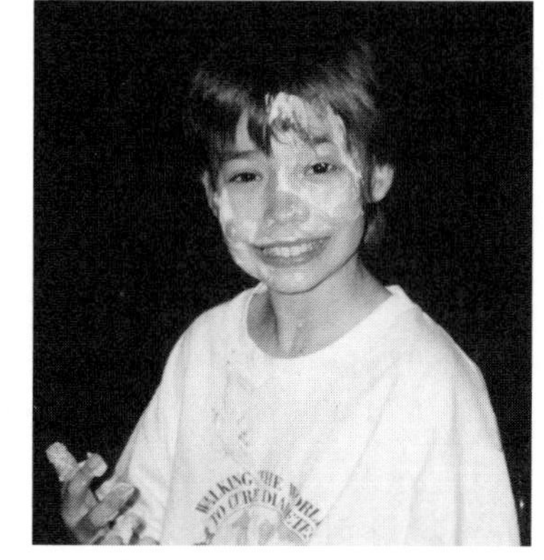
Cory Graham

Tip: When you're wearing a nightgown, clip your pump to the collar/neckline. *–Sophie Sheridan, age 9*

Tip: During sports you can disconnect your pump and use a syringe or an insulin pen to cover highs.

–Nick Brown, age 13

Tip: One nice thing about the pump is your lows don't tend to be as low when you are exercising.

–Emily Stahlman, age 10

Tip: If a lot of people ask me what my pump is, I just tell them that something inside of me doesn't work anymore, and this gives me medicine.

–Kelly Hrubeniuk, age 10

Tip: When you wear the pump, it just becomes routine.
–Mary Costello, age 21

Tip: I like the pump. It's so convenient.
–Brendan Black, age 19

Tip: The clip on the back of my Paradigm lets me spin my pump around, so I can get a better look at it without taking it off. *–James Neil, age 12*

Tip: On the pump, you can eat whenever you want, and there's a lot more freedom. *–Brandon Velilla, age 14*

Tip: When you don't feel well even if your blood sugar numbers are OK, test for ketones.
–Julia Halprin Jackson, age 18

Tip: When traveling with your pump, if you expect to make 3 site changes, carry 2 extra sets for backup. You take: 5 reservoirs, 5 infusion sites with tubing attached, an extra vial of insulin, and a package of syringes—just in case your pump malfunctions. *–Blair Ryan, age 16*

Tip: In case your pump breaks or malfunctions, you should keep a bottle of long-lasting insulin (like Lantus) and a bottle of fast-acting insulin (like Humalog) on hand. A daily injection of Lantus pretty much works as your basal rate, which is very much like being on the pump. You would also need to take shots of Humalog when you eat—just like you would bolus on the pump.
–Brandon Velilla, age 14

CHAPTER FOUR

Vacations, Camp, and Traveling around the World

Vacation

Virtually everyone we have talked to said they have had big lows both the night before and the first night of vacations, trips, moving, going off to college . . . etc. Vacations, trips, and big changes in routine are exciting. Excitement can lower blood sugars. Take a few moments the night before a big trip and make sure you test, snack, and maybe reduce your nighttime insulin. While on vacation, it's OK to lower your nighttime insulin dose, or your early morning basal rate, if you are seeing low numbers!

- It's easy to forget what you just ate, whether or not you tested, and how much insulin you just injected when your routine is interrupted. Take a logbook and write everything down.

Tip: Low blood sugars are common the night before a vacation starts (I'm always too excited to sleep before a big road trip), so be sure to test and eat a bedtime snack, just like you're already on vacation.

–Clare Rosenfeld, age 16

Tip: Know where your emergency supplies are and let someone know that lows happen during exciting times and changes in routine. (We recommend keeping your emergency supplies in your cooler. That way you can find them.) *–Brittany Brown, age 10*

Tip: Long car trips and lack of activity can lead to high blood sugars (usually during the day). Test often and take ketone testing strips on vacation. *–A.J. Fenner, age 18*

Keep your cool

At Bass Lake this summer, little Laura Valine's dad took her small black kit (containing her insulin) down to the dock and set it on a towel in the sun. When he gave Laura her dinner shot of 25/75, she immediately got very low. The heat had broken down the long-acting portion of the insulin, so it reacted very quickly. Laura's parents immediately took care of her low sugar. Then they threw away the overheated insulin and replaced it.

Tip: When you change your routine, especially on vacations, keep your insulin cool. Heat can ruin your short-acting insulin. Heat may also cause long-lasting insulin to work like short-acting insulin, resulting in a very low blood sugar episode. *–Diane, Laura Valine's mom*

Tip: Take extra insulin on vacation and keep it cool. *–Jessica Lopez, age 16*

Tip: When we drive down to Mexico, say for three days, I figure out how many needles and how much insulin I'm going to need. Then I pack extra needles and insulin. I keep my insulin in a cooler with an ice pack. I drink bottled water when we travel.

–Jessica Lopez, age 16

Grad night at Disneyland

Mike: When you visit theme parks, plan ahead. Check with big institutions like Disneyland—they may offer ways to make your vacation easier. During Grad Night at the *Magic Kingdom*, I carried my kit and snacks around all night. Four years later, when my brother Eric spent his Grad Night at Disneyland, Disney provided a central location where he could stash his kit and snacks. It made the evening go much more smoothly!

–Mike Brin, age 20

Tip: Make sure someone is with you when you are at a theme park and agree on a place to meet if you get split up! Carry money for snacks. *–Stephen Whitlock, age 16*

Tip: You can go to Disneyland's City Hall for a Guest Assistance pass (front of line). Little kids who get very excited often get low at theme parks.

–A.J. Fenner, age 18

Tip: On very hot days, kids can get low while waiting in lines. You may want to take advantage of the ability to go to the front of the line at theme parks.

–Ryan Ficke, age 17

Tip: I call my glucagon kit my "red shot" so my friends and family have "red" in their heads if an emergency arises. I keep my glucagon kit in my red canvas emergency bag.

–Mary Costello, age 21

Off to Camp

Bo: In July, while Spike traveled in Spain, I visited Julia Halprin Jackson, at Camp Conrad-Chinnock in Big Bear,

Where Is My Glucagon?

Brittany Brown and her family had just arrived in Las Vegas on vacation when, in the early morning hours, Brittany dropped to a severe low. Brittany was out and her parents were scrambling around, throwing things everywhere, looking for sugar and looking for her glucagon kit. (Away from home, in an unfamiliar place, living out of suitcases, they had no routine and didn't know where anything was.)

They put frosting between her cheek and gums, and she didn't wake up. They tried juice. They called 911. Brittany's dad finally found the glucagon kit and ripped it open, but he was so anxious he didn't notice the vial of glucagon powder when it flew out and rolled under the bed. He ended up injecting Brittany in the leg with just the liquid that comes in the syringe. Needless to say, the shot did nothing for her.

When the paramedics arrived, they put instant glucose gel in her cheek, and she came to in a matter of minutes.

Tip: When you are traveling, always have your frosting or glucose gel and glucagon in your cooler, where you can find it!

–Brittany Brown, age 10

Tip: Read the directions for using glucagon before you need to use it (page 253).

–Brittany Brown, age 10

What the Doc Says:

Review the directions on the Glucagon box every year so you'll know what to do when you need to do it. Christmas vacation is a good time; it's an exciting time for little kids, and it's right in the middle of flu season.

–Marc Weigensberg, MD

California. What an experience seeing Julia working with the kids in her cabin. It made me wish I'd gone to camp. She wrote me this letter so we could share her camp experience:

Dear Bo,

I love anything that involves being outside, especially sports like swimming, water-skiing, and hiking, so being a counselor-in-training (CIT) at Camp Chinnock was a natural. In July 2001 I packed my bag, flew to Southern California, and took a taxi to meet 100-plus excited kids, their parents toting sleeping bags, snacks, needles, and supplies, and counselors and staff members who were already chanting camp songs and making friends with the kids. Leaving parents behind in the parking lot, we boarded yellow school buses and were on our way to Camp Conrad-Chinnock.

Each day at camp was filled with exciting activities. Counselors and CITs led their cabins to the pool or on hikes with the naturalist. Kids were working on crafts, rock climbing, rappelling, and gold panning—they could even go mountain bike riding.

Camp food was great. We ate three meals a day in the raucous camp lodge, and snacks mid morning, mid afternoon, and before lights out.

Before each meal, the counselors and camp medical staff assisted the kids as they checked their blood sugars, drew up insulin shots, or discussed boluses on insulin pumps. Changes in insulin dosages, whether basal rate decreases or changes in long-lasting insulin like NPH, Lente, Ultralente, or Lantus, were discussed with the camp doctors. Generally, kids and doctors made about a 10% decrease on long-lasting insulin doses or basal rates.

- Excitement affects kids in different ways at camp. Some kids needed drastic decreases in insulin, while others needed more than they took at home because of all the adrenaline rushes or hormone changes.
- Supplies were provided for kids on injections for the duration of camp: insulin, needles, even testing kits. Pumpers were asked to bring reservoirs, sets, tape, and the tubing necessary for changing sites throughout the week.

The normality of it all amazed me—how these kids could do these wonderful things, stop briefly to make adjustments to their insulin dosages, take their own shots, and then continue their activities.

For someone who had been diagnosed just five months before, and who had been known to sometimes check more than 10 times a day, I found that camp was truly my first time to take a deep breath and relax. Camp was the first place I could see diabetes as just a minor adjustment to my schedule. I didn't have to stop and explain to anyone what anything meant. I never felt awkward checking my blood when other people were around.

Overall, I just loved the feeling of being a part of a team. To see the kids having so much fun, making friends, and taking part in all of the activities—all the while dealing with the frustration that diabetes sometimes provides—has helped me become not only a better diabetic, but a better human being.

–Julia Halprin Jackson, age 17

Tip: While caring for 6 to 8 year olds at Camp De Los Ninos, I sometimes have trouble keeping water down my kids during activities—and especially during high ketones. We had so much fun with water drinking contests. The kids and I would have water drinking contests to get re-hydrated, and I would always be left to cope with losing the contest. *–Mary Costello, age 21*

Tip: Go to diabetes camp. It's fun! ☺ *–Jenna Rohm, age 16*

Tip: I like going to diabetes camp because diabetes is normal there. Everybody is testing and taking insulin. I also really like meeting new friends.

–Megan Kaniasty, age 11

Tip: Attending camp has changed my life. Before camp I was an adolescent who was lost. At camp I discovered I'm not the only one, and then I turned my energy into being a mentor and helping other kids. I am loving what I am doing now. *–Ryan Martz, age 20*

Bo: A few months later, Julia shared exciting news. She was on the pump. I must say it was a revelation to me seeing this newly-diagnosed 17-year-old girl doing so well on the pump. The next time we hung out, she had it casually clipped to her bathing suit like it was the most natural thing in the world. I remember thinking, "I could do this."

A Teen Retreat

Bo: Growing up in Upper Ojai (also known as "the middle of nowhere"), every day was like camp. We have coyotes, bobcats,

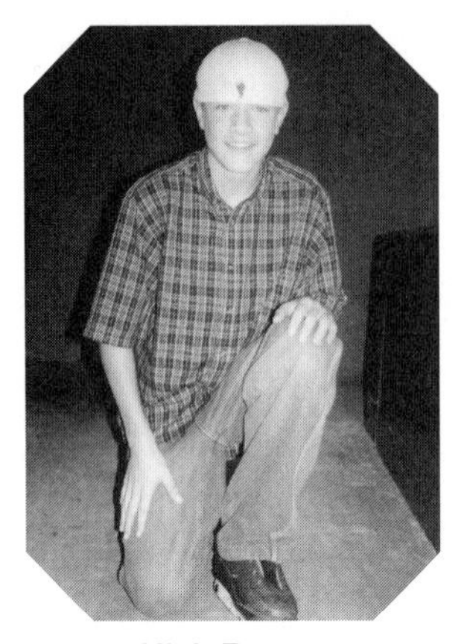

Nick Brown

deer, and even the occasional bear. When we felt like camping out, we walked about 100 yards into the wilderness—that's why we never went to diabetes camp. Spike and I did, however, go to a teen retreat at UCLA.

It was awesome. We met a bunch of great kids. We did skits, played games, and even learned a little about diabetes. It was really neat to meet so many up-beat kids who have diabetes just like us.

Tip: The Teen Retreat was awesome. I got to hang out with kids my own age who have diabetes too, and they didn't bug you about why you have to test.

–Nick Brown, age 13

Tip: I liked the teen retreat at UCLA and would recommend it. It was a lot of fun. I'd like to return next year as a counselor. *–Brandon Velilla, age 14*

Tip: I recently attended the teen retreat at UCLA, which I enjoyed and found relaxing. *–Brendan Black, age 19*

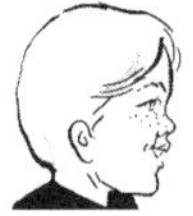

After hearing about diabetes camp, and after going to the PADRE weekend retreat, we definitely recommend camps and overnight retreats for kids with diabetes.

Traveling around the World

Spike and The Rhino

The glaring African sun beat down upon the bush and all its inhabitants. At the time, these included myself, four family members, and our armed tracker, Meshack. We had been out in the midday heat for roughly an hour and were eager to be back at our camp, poolside, with cold drinks all around. We must have been a little too eager, for none of us saw the two-ton, foot-long-horn-bearing rhino until we were no more than a dozen yards away.

The huge white rhino stood and sniffed the air. Upon catching the scent of the invaders of its territory, it gave a snort and stomped at the ground, veldt dust billowing up into the still air.

"When he charges," spoke our guide in his thick Zulu accent, "run for the rocks." With that he shouldered his rifle and signaled for us to be quiet. When he charges?!

Oh boy. I think my blood sugar dropped 50 points, instantly.

Mad thoughts raced through my mind. How could that peashooter of a gun stop that freight train of an animal if he didn't want to stop? How could I outrun an infuriated rhino? How would it feel to be impaled and trampled? Was I wearing clean underwear? We were paralyzed. We could barely breathe as we watched the rhino swing its head back and forth, dull eyes not quite focusing. The rifle was poised. We had each chosen the spot in the rocks we would run for. There was no breeze; the sweat built up. . . .

Luckily I didn't have to answer the questions running through my head, for the rhinoceros stomped in place and then just stared, allowing us to inch our way backwards. Meshack still stood rooted to the spot, facing down the rhino. The rest of us kept backing away until we were a hill away from the rhino. We didn't know if we were shaking from being low or from sheer terror, but Bo and I each ate a granola bar anyway. In fact, Jenny had one, too!

This story is more about not getting trampled by giant wild animals than it is about dealing with diabetes, but it touches on one of the most important points of this book: **Be prepared for anything, and you can do everything**. Simply by having a backpack stocked with food, Bo and I were able to trek for miles through the South African bush. We were even able to calm my sister down, and that's *never* easy.

- When traveling, always be prepared; you never know when an angry rhino will get between you and your camp!
- Keep your insulin kit on your person at all times: Insulin, syringes, meter, extra battery, test strips. Pumpers should carry syringes, in case their pump malfunctions.
- Carry a cooler or backpack with snacks that will last for at least 24 hours.
- Bring medications in case you become ill.
- Put your doctor's phone number in your kit.
- Before big trips to out-of-the-way places, get necessary inoculations.
- Carry Pepto Bismol. Begin taking tablets a few days before your trip to help avoid diarrhea. Note: Pepto Bismol turns stools black.
- Snack frequently the day before a big trip, and eat a nighttime snack including some protein. (Just the anticipation of a trip can cause severe low blood sugars.)
- Carry extra food on airplanes. You never want to run out of food.
- Carry a logbook and keep track of your sugars, dosages, and activities.

Tip: If you are new to traveling long distances, work out time zone changes and your insulin schedule with your doctor before you leave home. *–Mike Brin, age 20*

Tip: When you're traveling, check your sugars often.
–Alexie Milton, age 14

Tip: Carry a second set of everything in case your diabetes supplies are lost, stolen, or broken.
–Julia Halprin Jackson, age 18

The backpack

This is a list of what we carry when we are traveling around the country or around the world. When we are just hiking (like when we encountered our friend Mr. Rhinoceros), we carry our daypacks. Daypacks have the same stuff listed in the main body below, plus frosting and minus the book. Who reads when there are elephants and orangutans walking around?

If you're a parent traveling with a small child, carry an identical back-up backpack, just in case something gets broken, lost, or stolen.

The main body of the backpack contains:

- Insulin kit or pump and extra sites, tubing and vials
- Meter
- Gatorade
- Snacks packed in brown paper bags
- 1 box crackers
- 1 box cookies
- Jerky
- A whole box of granola bars
- Jacket
- Hat
- Book

The side pocket contains:

- Glucagon kit
- Ketostix
- Frosting
- Tylenol
- Imodium for diarrhea
- Neosporin and bandaids
- Compazine*, Phenergan, or Tigan for nausea
  (*Compazine is not for small children)
- Copy of *Symptoms*

The inside pocket contains:

- Passport
- Tickets
- Money
- Flattened insulin boxes with prescription label attached

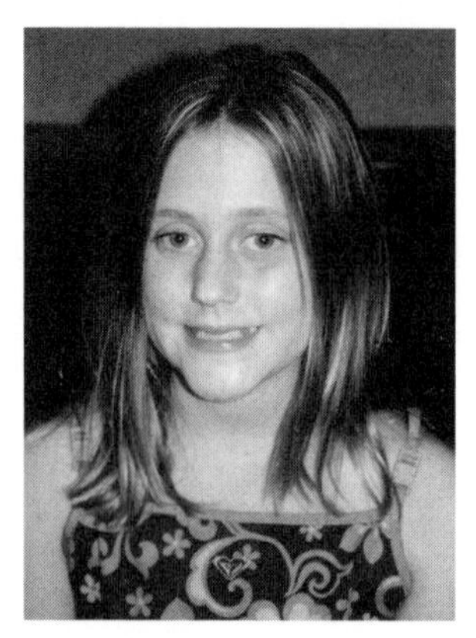

Brittany Brown

The large front pocket contains:

- Toothbrush
- Special medical supplies (such as asthma medication)
- Chapstick
- Deodorant
- Razor
- Swimmer's ear drops
- Sunscreen lotion
- Pens
- Small notebook

➠ **Note:** *Getting a Grip on Diabetes* devotes an entire chapter to traveling the globe.

Travel: Get Organized

Bo: When you travel, you need to be more organized. Carry two of everything, and be sure to wear your medical ID bracelet or necklace. It's a good idea to have your parents, friend, or sibling carry your back-up kit in case you lose your backpack. Spike and I always carry enough food for 24 hours in case we get stranded and keep our insulin supplies with us at all times.

Tip: Whenever I travel anywhere, I bring back-up insulin and needles. *–Herbert Larkin, age 17*

Tip: When you travel or backpack, pop your insulin vials into padded holders. *–Derrick Crowe, age 8*

Tip: Take a back-up bottle of insulin, syringes, or an insulin pen, and a change of tips for the pen.
–Nick Brown, age 13

Tip: Don't put extra insulin in your checked luggage. Carry it. Baggage compartments get too cold. Extreme cold and heat mess up your insulin. *–Clare Rosenfeld, age 16*

Tip: Don't put your expensive insulin in hotel refrigerators outside of your room. If you need to cool it down, ask for ice. Wrap your insulin in a plastic bag. Keep insulin from direct contact with the ice using a second baggie as a cushion. *–Clare Rosenfeld, age 16*

Tip: You can keep your insulin in the in-room refrigerator of your hotel or motel if they have one, just don't put it close to the freezer section. *–Clare Rosenfeld, age 16*

Tip: Put your ice pack in the hotel freezer.
–Ant Engeln, age 14

Tip: When traveling, take a photocopy of your passport, driver's license, and prescription for insulin and syringes. This will help you get what you need if your important papers and meds are lost or stolen. (Leave a second copy of these documents at home with someone available by phone.)
–Josh Halprin Jackson, Julia's brother

Tip: I always carry extra plastic baggies to use for protecting my insulin, meter, and pump. *–Clare Rosenfeld, age 16*

No food to be found in Johannesburg, South Africa

Bo: Be prepared. We can't emphasize this enough. No matter where you are going, have the essentials on hand (your kit—

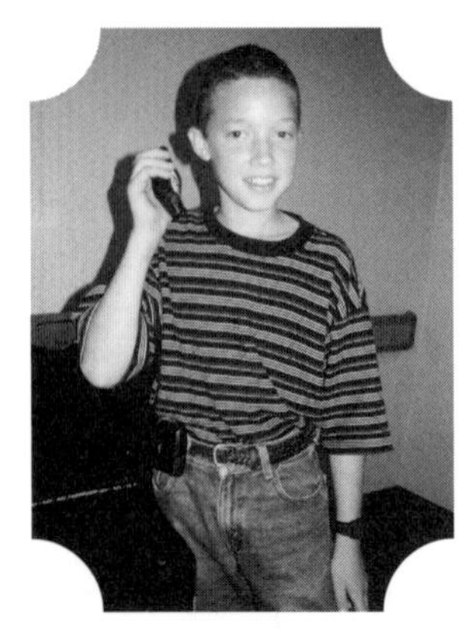

Brian Feinzimer

insulin and meter—and enough food to get by in a worst-case scenario). For example, if you are planing an hour-long bike ride, actually prepare to travel half an hour away from your departure point and get a flat tire. Now your half-hour return ends up taking three hours or more. This kind of potential delay means that you need to take Gatorade in a sports bottle, your insulin kit in a saddle on the bike, and enough granola bars to get you back home in case your blood sugar drops.

The customs in other areas and countries may be different. In some countries they take siestas in the afternoon, and all the stores are closed. In others you can't buy a bite to eat until noon, and dinner is served at 10:00 PM. You may run into a situation in a foreign country where you can't get bottled water. There are holidays where everything is closed for three days, odd hours, and strikes to consider. To make traveling smooth and safe, always prepare for the unexpected—develop the worst-case scenario.

A perfect example of a worst-case scenario happened when Spike and I were catching a flight from Johannesburg, South Africa, to California. We had no reason to expect a problem since on the 18-hour flight to Africa we had been served breakfast, lunch, and dinner; and the flight attendants handed out bottled water, soft drinks, and bags of nuts. Just before boarding the return flight, we discussed dumping from our backpacks the granola bars, nuts, and crushed crackers we had been hauling around for three weeks. In an abundance of caution, we decided to hang on to our basic snacks.

Good thing, since the unexpected happened. The airline support crew went on strike, right then and there. They didn't serve any food or refreshments at all. This could have been really bad.

What saved Spike and me was being prepared. We each had our own backpack with a bottle of Gatorade, six granola bars, Cheez-Its, and beef jerky. Please prepare for the unexpected. You can do anything you want to do as long as you are well prepared.

- Give yourself at least 2 weeks to work with your insurance company to order extra supplies you will need on your trip.
- Whenever traveling away from a source of food (home, restaurants or grocery stores) carry at least a 24-hour supply of food.

Foreign lands, foreign languages

Mary Costello just returned from studying in Europe. She discovered that being in countries where you can't speak the language presented a few challenges. The first thing Mary did when she stepped off the plane was to ask the travel people for the local phone number equivalent to 911. She came up with the following tips to make things run more smoothly:

- Ask airport or hotel personnel for the local 911 number. Give that number to all the people you are traveling with. If you're going to need emergency services, your friends are the ones who are going to make the call. You can also find that information at: http://ambulance.eire.org/Numbers/Index.htm.
- In the language of every country you are going to visit, learn how to pronounce:
    - I have diabetes.
    - I need sugar.

Write down the phone number of the local ER and the following phrases in the language of the country you are visiting. Have the information in your kit, or give it to your travel buddy. In an extreme emergency, things will go more smoothly. If you have a severe low blood sugar episode, your friends will be able to communicate. If you pass out, they can say:

TRANSLATIONS

English	Spanish	French
Mary has diabetes.	Mary tiene la diabetes.	Mary a le diabète.
She needs sugar/glucose.	Ella necesita azúcar.	Elle a besoin du sucre.
She is in insulin shock.	Ella está en el golpe de insulina.	Elle est dans le choc d'insuline.

- You can go to http://www.freetranslation.com/ to get translations in more languages for any phrase you want.

On a lighter note, in restaurants you are going to want to order sugar-free drinks. When I visited Europe, I was served a real Coke because they didn't understand me. I drank about 60 grams of carbohydrate before I thought to double-check if it was sugar free. (Their Coke Lite tastes like real Coke, so I didn't think anything of the more sugary taste.) American expressions are used in many countries. In Europe they generally say Coke Lite.

Tip: In the language of every country you are going to visit, learn how to pronounce:

TRANSLATIONS

English	Spanish	French
I want a diet soda.	Quiero una "coca lite."	Je veux une soude "lite."

When it comes to watching what you eat, things can get tricky. Since you eat out a lot and you're eating foods that are very different from what you normally eat, counting carbs can be a challenge. Keep the following in mind:

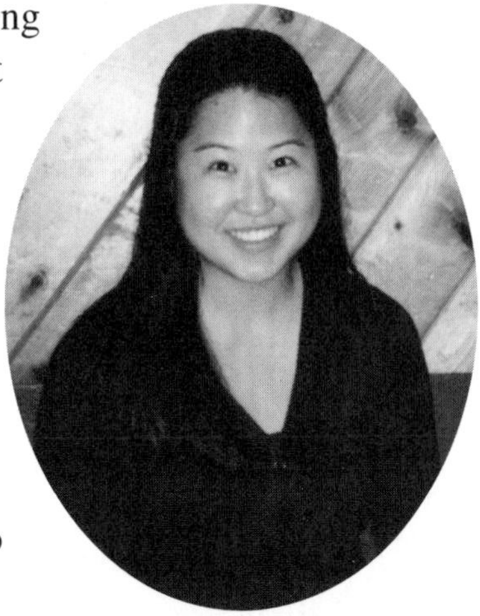

- Do some measuring before you leave home to travel, so you can eyeball serving sizes.
- Look up foods before you leave or buy a cheap nutrition book when you get there (if it's in English). Try *The Diabetes Carbohydrate and Fat Gram Guide*, 3rd edition (ADA, 2004).
- You'll find good carb-counting links on the insulin pumpers' website at www.insulin-pumpers.org.

Jennifer Park

Tip: You can dip a Diastick strip into a soda to check for sugar if you're not sure it is diet soda. Compare to the color chart after 30 seconds. *–Gabriel Fieger, age 8*

Traveling by air

Don't worry, your pump will not set off security alarms in airports. I found it easiest to place my pump in a pocket, to avoid being held up answering questions. If security people do ask you questions, explain its function and do not remove your pump—even if asked. Just keep explaining that it's a life-sustaining medical device. Ask to talk to a superior if necessary.

- Carry the box your insulin comes in with all prescription info on it. This is what security uses to prove you have diabetes.

- If traveling for a long period of time, you may want to call the medical department of the airline you're flying. They can approve more baggage for your supplies.
- Watch out for lows in planes and airports, especially when you're about to land. For some reason (excitement maybe), I was low 90% of the time when landing in an airport.
- Most airlines will let you take a cooler on board. Call ahead and find out.
- Stay hydrated (which may mean avoiding excessive caffeine intake). Staying hydrated helps you avoid highs and also helps to avoid jet lag symptoms.
- Try to get up and get the blood flowing as much as possible during flights; it's better for your circulation.

"God gave those of us with the most character the biggest challenges . . . and you can take that as a compliment." (A friend gave me this quote and I thought it might be nice to tell others the same.) Bon voyage!

–Mary Costello, age 21

Tip: Carry a letter of medical necessity when traveling, especially when traveling by air. *–Jennifer Park, age 21*

Tip: Wear a medical ID bracelet or necklace. It helps at security and will also insure you'll be treated properly in an emergency. *–Ryan Ficke, age 17*

Tip: If you have a pump and are worried it might break while traveling, you can call your pump company, and borrow an extra travel pump that you return when you arrive home. *–Clare Rosenfeld, age 16*

Tip: Always keep your supplies on board with you. That way you know the temperatures your supplies are exposed to, and you won't have your supplies lost or damaged.

–Mary Costello, age 21

Spring break, bellyache, and glucagon

Spike: Spring break in Mexico is a rite of passage for many college students. Although week-long beer binges and mornings where you find yourself asking, "What happened?" aren't exactly my style, I wasn't going to let my last spring break as a college student go by without a trip to a Mexican party town. After heated deliberations with my girlfriend, Vanessa, we decided to join my fraternity brothers and her sorority sisters in Mexico—just not in the same beer-bingeing party town where they were going. It was a sacrifice, but it was a good decision.

To enjoy the true flavor of Mexico, we decided to rough it once in awhile for dinner. Vanessa was a champ and ate at all the little taco stands right along with me. She stopped short of imbibing the water, though. She warned me not to drink it, and I think I said something along the lines of, "Oh, stop being a girl. I've been to Mexico so many times. I eat everything. I never get sick in Mexico." Famous last words.

By day four I couldn't even get out of bed to go and get a massage, much less hit the beach. It was rough. I wasn't throwing up, but my stomach was tied in more knots and hurt in more places than I thought it had, and I had just taken an anatomy class. I let my sugar run a little high, because I was expecting to throw up at any moment, and my appetite for tacos and salsa picante had diminished markedly. I didn't sleep much that last night, as the cramping had gotten progressively worse, and my fears of the long, hot flight home in the morning started setting in.

Breakfast was a piece of white bread without the crust and some Gatorade I bought at a little tienda down the street from the hotel. Sipping warm Gatorade (no more ice) was about the only thing my poor little tummy could handle. Vanessa had to carry both of our duffel bags through the lobby to the taxi and through the airport. I know each one weighed more than she does, but she managed to carry them—on top of playing nurse and finding me real 7-Up, and even a straw to drink it with.

Despite her TLC, I lost it at the airport and had to run outside and throw up. No one paid me any heed, as a lot of dumb American kids do the same thing the last day of Spring Break at the airport, but usually for a different reason. Once I got it all out of my system, I went back inside and checked my sugar. It was 80. A little low for getting ready to fly, and a lot low considering I might not be keeping anything else down. I ate what I could and checked again 20 minutes later—65. I hadn't taken much insulin that morning in anticipation of such a problem, but evidently it was still too much since I was eating almost nothing.

I decided I had better take a glucagon injection. I had a glucagon kit in my insulin kit and just took it right there at the airport. Although Vanessa had been given the lecture about how glucagon was like the opposite of insulin and how she should give it to me if I were ever really out of it, she had never seen it in action, so I walked her through the steps. You inject the liquid out of the syringe and into the bottle with the little tablet. Then you shake it until the tablet is totally dissolved. Then you fill the syringe back up and take a shot wherever you want. I used my butt, as I do for all of my insulin injections. The syringe was a little bigger than my B-D Ultra-Fines, but it really didn't hurt, and I knew it would make me feel a lot better and a lot less worried about my sugars. I took the entire dose.

I kept sipping real small doses of Gatorade and 7-Up, enough to get a few calories in me but not enough to make me sick again. I tested about 25 minutes after the glucagon, and my sugar was back up to 110. I tested 2 more times on the plane, and I was 135 and 185. It was really nice to see my sugars coming up even though I couldn't eat much, and the flight was a lot better without worrying about dropping blood sugar. Plus, since I was still kind of sick, Vanessa actually let me have the window seat.

Tip: Fifteen minutes after injecting glucagon, eat some sugar or carbs, and eat some again 15 minutes later. This will help stop your blood sugar from dropping again, and help keep your sugars level. *–Jackie Teichman, PADRE*

CHAPTER FIVE

Sick Days, Accidents, and Surgery

When You Are Sick

You'll need help when you are sick. Get your mom or dad to help balance your insulin intake and calories. You can do this—just get organized and:

- Test your sugar often.
- Drink lots of fluids.
- Keep taking insulin.
- Call your doctor if things aren't going well.

Ketones

What are ketones? If you don't have enough insulin in your system, sugar (glucose) can't get into your cells. Starved for energy, your body starts to break down stored fat. A by-product of burning fat is ketones. Your body tries to get rid of the ketones in the urine, leading to dehydration. You usually see high blood sugar with ketones. The body tries to get rid of the sugar (glucose) through the urine, which again leads to dehydration. So it's a double whammy. The combination of dehydration and ketones is ketoacidosis, and it can make you feel awful.

Test for ketones

We need to test for ketones when we are sick. High ketones mean you need more fast-acting insulin, more often. Check with your doctor the first few times you have ketones until you get the hang of handling it. High ketones combined with dehydration leads to ketoacidosis. If you have "large ketones" combined with the symptoms of ketoacidosis (DKA), call your doctor right away.

Symptoms of ketoacidosis

- Nausea and vomiting
- Rapid, deep breathing
- Loss of appetite
- Abdominal pain
- Weakness
- Visual disturbances
- Sleepiness

When you are on the pump, ketones require immediate action (page 217).

Tip: If you test positive for ketones, drink lots of water or sugar-free liquids, then drink some more.

–Scott Shiebler, age 15

Tip: If you feel queasy, or you're vomiting, check for ketones. Check even if you don't have high blood sugar.

–Scott Shiebler, age 15

Tip: When you are sick or running high blood sugar (240 or above) several times in a row, test for ketones. You'll want to catch ketones as they are first developing (mild or moderate) when they are easier to get rid of.

–Scott Shiebler, age 15

Tip: When you have "large" ketones, keep the fluids going. Watch yourself if you throw up. Test often. Make sure to contact your doctor if the ketones don't come down and you are vomiting, or if you can't keep liquids down.
–Scott Shiebler, age 15

Tip: Water with Nu-Salt is good to help restore potassium levels if you have ketones. (See Nu-Salt at www.nusalt.com). *–Mary Costello, age 21*

Tip: Keep a bottle of ketone test strips in your house. Take them with you when you travel. *–Scott Shiebler, age 15*

The flu

Sometimes you vomit when you have the flu. This is the time a lot of kids with diabetes get into trouble. We have insulin in our system, we eat, we vomit, and our blood sugar drops.

- Drink your calories with sugary drinks like real 7-Up, Gatorade, or ginger ale. Only drink a little at a time when you are nauseated (*very* little—like 1 teaspoon every 5 minutes).

If you vomit once, alert your family or roommate to stand by—or call someone and let them know you may need help. There is that ten minutes or so after you throw up when you feel OK. Set up your back-up help then. If you vomit twice, call and have someone stay with you while you are sick.

- Spread out your fast-acting insulin. Take what you need for the carbs you are taking in with a small dose (if you are injecting, say 2 units, every two hours. If you are pumping, you can take super small boluses more frequently).
- Call your doctor if things get out of control. Test your blood sugar and ketones right before you make the call.
- Make sure you have a glucagon kit in your diabetes drawer or cooler (page 19).
- It's OK to go to the emergency room if you need fluids. The ER is our friend. Take your kit when you go to the ER. Take your packed cooler too.
- Get a flu shot—every year.

–James Neil, age 12

Accidents

Bo tangles with a mountain bike

This past summer I purchased a high-quality mountain bike with some of the money I had made waiting tables. At first I was really into going on long rides deep into the mountain trails around my house, but things changed part way through summer.

Back when we were little kids, Spike and I had used our dad's tractor to build jumps for our dirt bikes. Naturally, I decided to use an *old* jump with my new mountain bike. The first few times going over the jump I was just trying to get a feel for it; but when my friend Jake came over, he challenged me to clear the jump. I got going about twice as fast as before and cleared the jump—by a lot actually. Unfortunately, when I landed, the bike collapsed underneath me, and the bike seat slammed into the small of my back, lacerating my kidney.

While my mom got the car, Jake grabbed my kit and cooler (packed and ready to go), and we headed for the emergency room. I tested my blood on the way and carbed-up (drank a little Gatorade), expecting that such a traumatic experience would lower my sugar. At the ER, between CAT scans, I tested my blood sugar frequently. It was nice to be able to have all the things I needed right with me. It was also really nice to have my mother there, someone who knew me and knew how to help me with my diabetes.

I spent a couple of nights in the hospital, a week flat on my back, and a month of watching my friends mountain bike and surf.

- Blood sugars tend to spike up right after an accident, and then bottom out. After an accident, sip Gatorade if you can.
- If you need to be taken to the hospital for a broken leg or stitches, take your insulin kit and take your cooler.
- Tell all the medical staff that you have diabetes.
- When you're in the ER, check your sugar during treatment, stitches, and between CAT scans.
- Bring your cooler filled with snacks, so they will be handy. Snack when you need carbs.
- Make sure your mom or dad also keeps track of your blood sugars and insulin intake. Write everything down. *You and your parents are the experts on your diabetes.*

Surgery

Surgery is a big deal for anyone, and with diabetes it can be a little trickier. Just like everything else, preparation is the key. Be sure and take your kit and cooler to the hospital. If you're organized and prepared, you can handle any challenges that surgery throws your way.

Blood sugar trends

An important concept we *just* learned (from Steven Whitlock and Clare Rosenfeld when they sent tips for this book) is the importance of determining your "blood sugar trends." You do this by testing your blood sugar several times in a row before events like surgery, an intense sports event, or giving a speech. That way you can see if your sugars are dropping or rising—see the trend. Once you know the direction your sugar is heading, you can better adjust your insulin and carb intake.

Tip: Check your blood sugar several times during the hours before surgery to see if you are dropping—to see the trend. *–Stephen Whitlock, age 16*

Tip: Check your blood sugar again right before surgery. *–Stephen Whitlock, age 16*

Tip: Have your mom or dad monitor your diabetes during your stay in the hospital. Mom or Dad should always double-check the amount of insulin nurses give you. *–Samantha McGuigan, age 8*

Wisdom teeth

Oral surgery is a special case, because (1) you are put under anesthesia, and (2) it's mouth surgery, so it's difficult to eat afterward.

Jennifer Ogden had her wisdom teeth removed and learned a lot about how to handle the ups and downs of oral surgery.

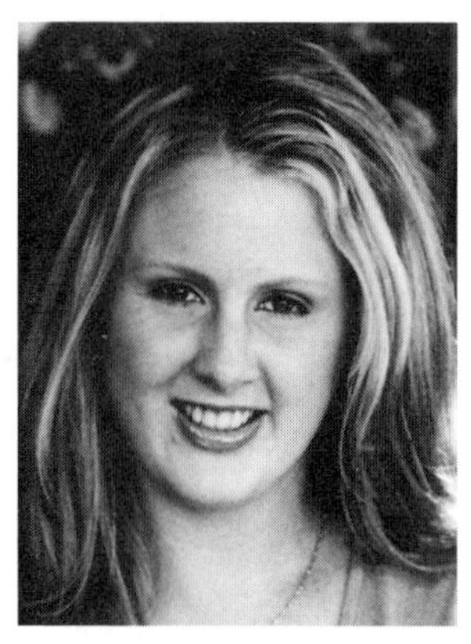

Jennifer Ogden

> Hi Spike and Bo, here's my surgery saga, hope it helps!
>
> Before surgery I was nervous, and my sugar began to drop. (This was my first oral surgery, after all.)
>
> - Nerves and anxiety can cause lower sugars.

Dr. Tim Flannery is a pediatric endocrinologist. This is what he had to say.

It's all about attitude. The oral surgeon needs to have a good attitude and work with you. Oral surgery only lasts about an hour, so check blood sugar before surgery. Have someone check your blood sugar every hour during and after surgery. The oral surgeon should be involved in the entire process.

Arrange to be the first patient in the morning. Since you are fasting the night before surgery, this is important.

Plan ahead. Have plenty of liquid carbohydrates on hand for after your surgery. For the next couple of days, you will be drinking your carbs instead of eating them. Things like Gatorade, juice, and shakes work really well for this.

After your surgery, take in your carbohydrates, and then inject to cover what you have to drink.

–Tim Flannery, MD

My mom tested me right there on the gurney—I was only 70—so she told the doctor my sugar was dropping. His nurse put me on a 5% glucose IV drip to keep me from getting any lower. As it turned out, the IV wasn't set up right, and I wasn't getting any glucose. The doctors and nurses were busy with the surgery and post-op and didn't notice the problem. My mom had to point it out to them and have it fixed.

- No one knows how to handle your diabetes as well as you and your parents. Make sure your mom or dad is with you the whole time pre-surgery and post-surgery to check your sugars and communicate with the medical staff.

- Check your blood sugar several times during the hours before oral surgery, so you can see the *trend.* Check again right before surgery.
- If the surgeon and staff aren't cooperative, don't use them. You call the shots. *–Jennifer Ogden, age 19*

Spike: My diabetes expert, my mom, drove up to Palo Alto to be with me when I had elbow surgery in college. Boy, was I grateful!

The ER and hospitals

We view the ER as our friend. It's a place to go to get your body back into balance. Grab your kit and your cooler on the way to the ER or have a family member bring your kit and cooler to you.

Tip: When you go to the hospital, make sure your parents are in charge. *–Samantha McGuigan, age 8*

Tip: Take your insurance card. Let your parents or friend deal with signing in and using your insurance card. If you can't find your card, have the hospital call your parents. It will save insurance hassles later on.
–Jennifer Ogden, age 19

Insurance

Jennifer has discovered that life is a lot less complicated if you stay on top of your health insurance. All insurance companies operate a little bit differently. The following general tips from Jennifer should help.

- Order the max diabetes supplies at one time. For example, for the same co-pay amount, you can get the maximum, 200 test strips instead of 100. This will cut your costs. (To think of all the money we wasted buying 100 strips at a time before we talked to Jennifer. *–Spike*)

- Blue Cross covers a maximum of 200 strips a month on one prescription. If the pharmacy declines any supplies, ask the pharmacy to call your insurance company to get an override.
- If your pharmacy denies strips or insulin, phone the 800 number on your insurance card. There is an override code that pharmacists can type in when ordering your supplies, so you get all that is allowed on your policy.
- Make sure your insurance is in place when you graduate from college. It's important not to let your insurance coverage lapse.
- In California keep your insurance up if there is a time between school and a job, even if you have to pay more for a COBRA Insurance plan. If you let your health insurance lapse for 2 or 3 months, companies can sometimes deny insurance.

–Jennifer Ogden, age 19

Tip: Don't be afraid to fight for what you need—more strips, different brands, etc. There is always someone higher-up to talk to. With Kaiser I have had success asking another doctor to write the prescription. I keep trying until I finally get what I need. I've also called member services for help. *–Mary Costello, age 21*

Doctors

General Practitioner (GP)

Everybody gets sick once in a while and needs a smart, friendly GP. Your GP needs to agree to see you the same day you call for ordinary problems like a cold, the flu, poison oak, or a sore throat. Since sugars can be a little trickier when you are sick, kids with diabetes need to be a little bit more careful and to stay on top of illnesses.

Endocrinologist, pediatric endocrinologist

Diabetes specialists—endocrinologists—are MDs who have two additional years of schooling in their field. It is their job to be up to date on the latest treatments available for managing diabetes. Your endocrinologist should inspire you with confidence and be able to guide you through anything. There are many brilliant endocrinologists out there. Find one!

- It's a good idea to write non-urgent questions down and to take your list with you when you go to see your doctor.

It's OK to change doctors

Bo: Going to a specialist can make all the difference in the world. This might be one of the simplest steps you can take to make a big difference in the way you feel every day. When Jessica, 18, was

Eye Doctors

Dr. Roger Phelps is an optometrist and a certified diabetes educator (CDE). Here are his recommendations:

Make sure you have a yearly dilated eye exam by an optometrist or ophthalmologist familiar with diabetes. If you should need treatment, ask to be referred to a retinal specialist. Retinal specialists have special training and expertise when it comes to the proper treatment of eye problems related to diabetes.

–Roger Phelps, OD, FAAO, CDE

first diagnosed at age 10, she went to her regular pediatrician. He started her on a super-strict diet that didn't work. When her numbers started skyrocketing, he put her on an enormous amount of Humalog (more than I was taking, and she weighs at least 50 pounds less than me). Her bouncing sugars and constant morning lows affected her schoolwork and her social life and left Jessica feeling tired and sick all the time. Jessica got back to feeling well because she had the courage to get a second opinion and began working with a specialist who knew what he was doing.

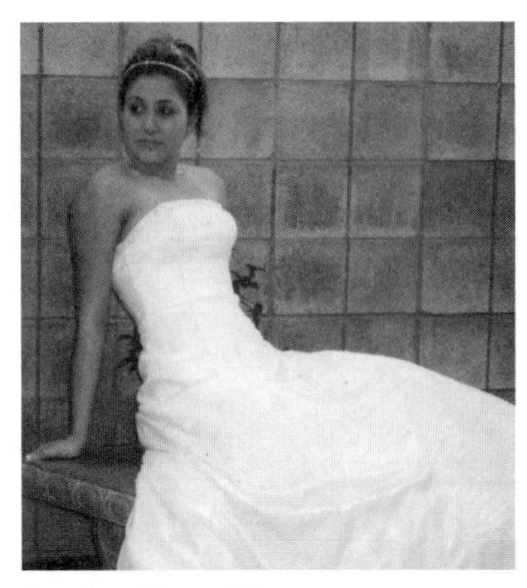

Jessica Stogsdill

Jessica: About the time life began to feel out of control, I switched to an endocrinologist who specializes in diabetes. He adjusted my insulin dose down to around 35 units per day and my glucose levels immediately leveled off where they were supposed to be. I am happy to say I got back on track in school and with my friends.

- See an endocrinologist!

–Jessica Stogsdill, age 18

➠ **Note:** Never worry about getting a second opinion. If your diabetes is out of control and you don't have confidence in your doctor, you may need to change doctors. You and your doctor need to be a good fit.

Tip: It's so important to feel comfortable with your doctor. If you can't tell your doctor anything and everything—change doctors. *–Mary Costello, age 21*

Tip: Diabetes care is constantly changing. If your doctor doesn't keep up, you may need to look for one who does. *–Mary Costello, age 21*

Girl Stuff

Hormones and periods

Although Bo and I like to consider ourselves experts on all things diabetes, while gathering tips for this book, we quickly realized there were some diabetes-related experiences that we had never had . . . and will never have in the future. We like to call these experiences Girl Stuff. Boys, feel free to skip this section. . . .

We have known Jenna Rinaldi since she was 14 years old. She moved away a couple of years ago, but we still keep in touch via e-mail.

> Hey Bo and Spike,
>
> I'll tackle the girl stuff for you. Sometimes it can be kind of frustrating when your blood sugar goes up for what seems like no reason at all. I notice that right before I start my period, my sugars surge (due to hormone fluctuations), and I get huge food cravings for sweet things like candy (more hormone fluctuations). I don't get too moody. I just get mad at my brother every once in a while, but that doesn't seem to affect my sugars. During my period, I take extra insulin just to cover what my hormones are doing.
>
> If you have trouble figuring out hormone fluctuations then it is important to get help from your doctor. I have always found that doctors are willing to help.

- Everyone's body reacts differently, but lots of girls notice their blood sugars go up right before their periods. You need to know your own body, and you need to know what to expect.

- Blood sugars tend to rise each month right before your cycle. You'll need to adjust your insulin a little to handle the highs.

–Jenna Rinaldi, age 18

Girl Stuff and the Pump

Because I am an athlete, my periods aren't on a 28-day cycle, but more of a four- to six-week cycle. My blood sugars tend to go higher the week before my special friend arrives.

Sometimes the difference in my blood sugars is slight, sometimes more dramatic. I may be having sugars in the 100s and see a slight elevation to, say the 200s, showing up for no reason. Sometimes I get wildly swinging sugars or really high sugars. This typically occurs the week before my period. It may take me a while to realize why my sugars are high, but once I do, I just increase my background insulin (my basal dose).

If you're on a long-lasting insulin, try increasing your long-lasting insulin a little bit from the moment you notice the high sugars (usually about 5–7 days before your period). Then just resume your normal dose the day your period starts.

I'm on the pump, so what works best for me is to increase my basal 0.2 from the time I notice high, erratic blood sugars until the day my period starts. The day it starts, I resume my normal basal.

–Mary Costello, age 21

Tip: That time of the month can affect your blood sugars. It is different for everyone, so test often to figure out how it affects you.

–Clare Rosenfeld, age 16

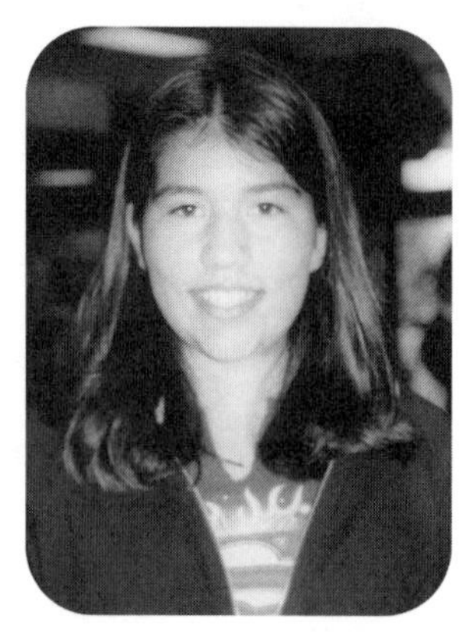

Alexie Milton

Tip: Tell your gynecologist you have diabetes.

–Jennifer Ogden, age 19

➠ **Note:** If you are going on the pill, ask your doctor about taking birth control with the lowest hormone dose. The pill may make your blood sugars run a little higher.

➠ **Note:** When estrogen and progesterone levels are high, insulin doesn't work as well and the liver releases more glucose into your bloodstream—so you see high blood sugars. If you see this pattern developing, adjust your insulin.

Growth Spurts

When you are growing, growth hormones and sex hormones interfere with the delivery of insulin. This kind of insulin resistance happens during puberty. You'll need a little extra insulin during growth spurts. Carry extra food when you are taking extra insulin. Once the growth spurt stops, you'll probably crash a little, and you'll need to lower your insulin dose then.

Tip: Hormones released during puberty and growth spurts can wreak havoc on blood sugars, causing them to soar.

–Rahwa, age 20

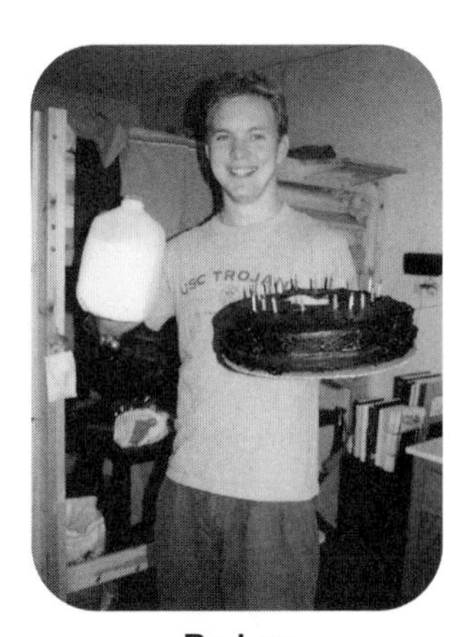

Bo Loy

The morning Bo didn't want to wake up

My first night back at college, junior year, I went to bed thinking it was going to be just like any other night. I had taken my short-acting Regular insulin a few hours earlier, for dinner, and 15 units of long-acting NPH about 1:30 AM (that's the earliest I go to bed at college).

My girlfriend, Rae, came by at some ridiculously early hour (OK, it was 8:00 AM). She tried to wake me up, but I just rolled over. I didn't get up. She thought I was just being lazy so she tugged at my arm, and I rolled onto the floor. Rae says I tried to talk to her, but I wasn't making any sense and was acting strange. Then when I gave her a blank stare, she started to cry. Scared, she called my mom, who guided her through what to do to get my sugars back up. Rae put frosting all around my gums, poured regular Coke into my mouth with a spoon, and tried to get me to drink some Gatorade. I remained unresponsive and unhelpful. When she would try to give me a spoonful of Coke, I'd say "No," and push her hand away. She wanted to use glucagon, but since I had just moved in the night before, she couldn't find my glucagon kit (it was still in my cooler in my car). After 15 minutes, when I hadn't come around, she called 911.

- Always put your glucagon kit in your diabetes drawer or your cooler as soon as you move in!

Moments after Rae got off the phone with the 911 operator, I started to wake up. Even in my groggy state, I knew something was up. Seeing the frosting and can of real Coke knocked some sense back into my head, so I started to follow Rae's directions. I drank all of the soda and a glass of orange juice and ate a granola bar.

- Keep your cooler packed with short-acting food in your room at college so everyone can find it.

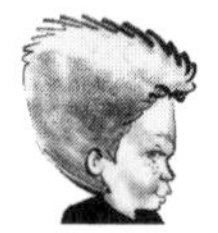

Great tip, Bo, but my experience has shown me that once your college friends know where to find your food, they will try to eat it. In addition to telling your friends where your cooler is, you may want to tape a note to it that reads "This is my emergency food only. This is not for you to eat, ______" and you can fill in the blank with your cheapest/hungriest friend's name. *–Spike*

By the time the paramedics arrived, I was feeling fine, and they asked me to test with my own test kit. I complied. My blood sugar was 193. Two granola bars and another glass of OJ later, I tested again, and I was 138. It didn't make sense. How could I go from 193 to 138 in 30 minutes, having done nothing but eat? We surmised that there was spilled Coke on my arm when I took my blood test.

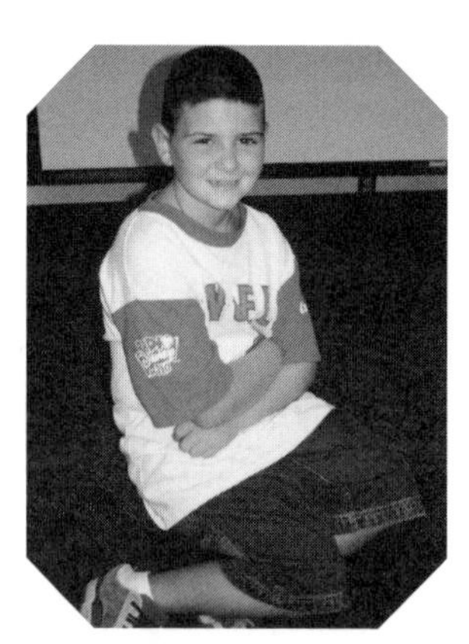

Jake Burnette

So what did I learn? If you feel really low and you test, and it doesn't show that you are low, test again at a different site. (Or eat food first and test later. It is better to be high for a while than to go lower.)

So now the question is, why did I have really low blood sugar on what seemed to be a normal night? I have a few guesses.

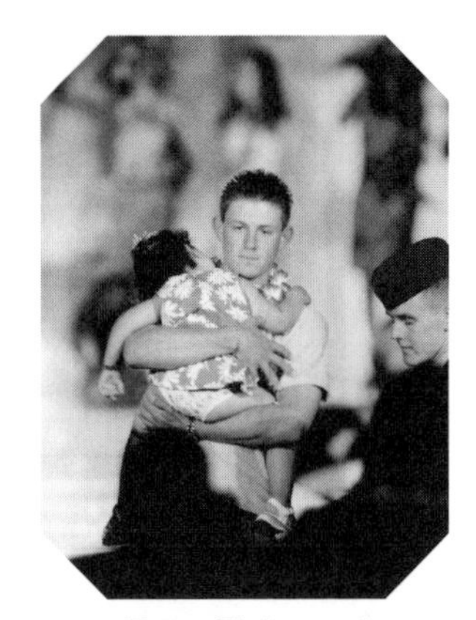
Ryan Ficke and Sarah Dorsey

- For one thing, I had been really sick the week before and had lost about 10 pounds. Losing that much weight probably depleted my body of all of its stored sugar (glycogen).
- My liver, which normally stores extra sugar to help me wake up in the morning, was probably also low on reserves.
- It had been an exciting few days getting back into the college routine, moving from home into my fraternity house. Excitement is a form of stress, albeit a good kind. Stress can cause wild blood sugar fluctuations.

I ran my 911 episode by Marc Weigensberg, MD, who explained what seems most probable. This low blood sugar episode occurred after a huge growing stage. During puberty, and when you are going through big growth spurts, you tend to develop some *insulin resistance* due to growth hormones. Once puberty is over, however, *insulin sensitivity* comes back.

Since I had just finished growing, there were fewer growth hormones in my body to interfere with insulin. I was still on the same NPH dosage, so what seemed to be a normal dose was actually an overdose.

I contacted my doctor the next day, and we worked out a regimen that would be more appropriate. I stopped using NPH at night and switched to Ultra Lente. It has less of a kick 6 to 8 hours after you take it.

Now that I am pumping, I am not taking any long-lasting insulin at all and feel even more secure that I won't have another morning like that one.

CHAPTER SIX

Cool Gadgets and Toys

Bo: Everybody has a favorite toy for handling diabetes—personal trackers, watches with multiple alarms, new testing toys. . . . Derrick Crowe, 8 years old, knows more about cool gadgets and toys that go along with diabetes than Spike and I put together. Derrick is our official Gadget Kid.

> Bo,
>
> It was very nice talking with you. I want you to know I love the new drink Propel because it tastes good, it is good for you, and the carbs are low (3 grams of carbs per 8 oz). Another good thing is that I feel like the other kids with my sports drink.
>
> Everyone in my family loves my watch with four timers. It reminds me when to eat even when I'm busy playing. We got you and Spike watches in case you get real busy. I know you are big and in college but you might be able to use it.
>
> Have fun surfing.
>
> Derrick

As you can see, Derrick loves his Fossil watch with four timers. He programs it for 10:00 AM (morning snack), 11:30 AM (when his NPH should kick in), 12:00 noon (lunch), and 3:00 PM (afternoon snack). Derrick loves the alarm system because when it goes off, he knows it's time for a snack or just an awareness check. Talk about being proactive, Derrick even wrote to Fossil and requested they make a watch with more than 4 alarms, because he could use two more—one alarm for dinner and one alarm for bedtime snack. Having all of those reminders is great for big kids too!

Tip: Having a watch with an alarm is good when other kids are over, and you lose track of time. When the alarm goes off, you know it's time for a snack.
–Derrick Crowe, age 8

Tip: If it's an important tool, have an extra one for back-up.
–Ryan Martz, age 20

New home A1C test

Spike and I first saw the Metrika A1C Now home meter at the ADA National Convention in San Francisco last summer and fell in love with it. It's easy to use and much more convenient than going into the doctor's office. You prick your finger or arm, put a drop of blood in a tube, shake it and wait 8 minutes.

Tip: The very best part about the A1C Now is—not poking your veins. *–Derrick Crowe, age 8*

Tip: The disposable A1Cs are heat sensitive, and they have a short shelf life of six months. No need to stock up on more than you can use. *–Derrick Crowe, age 8*

Tip: I use the Metrika one-time, home-use A1C meter to help get my A1C down. When I make changes in food or exercise to bring my daily sugars down, I can see it on the A1C. I recommend checking your A1C at home to everybody. I like to use the A1C meter often so I can watch my A1C averages come down (8.9 to 5.6).

–Chris Cisneros, age 14

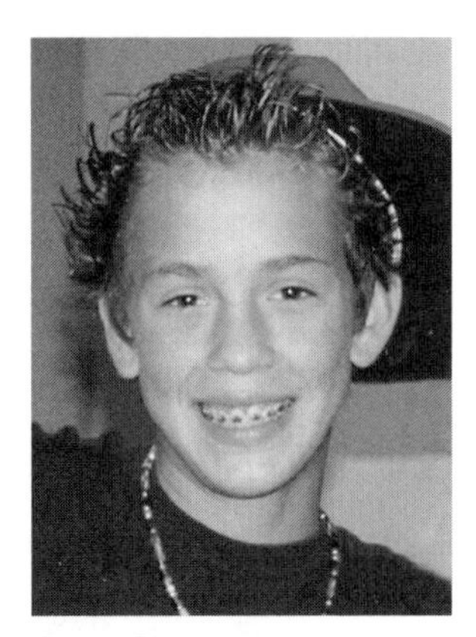

Chris Cisneros

Meters and arm pricks and finger pricks

There are great new tools for checking your blood sugar. Some new meters, Life Scan's One Touch Ultra and One Touch UltraSmart, and the FreeStyle by TheraSense need so little blood that you can test using the top of your arms. They are easy to use and way more comfortable than older meters.

- Rub the top of your forearm briskly before pricking. This will bring blood to the surface, so you only have to prick once.
- Prick your finger on the side of your finger, not the tip. It feels better.

It's a good idea to test your meter for accuracy about once a month or when you think your blood sugar reading is not right. The way to do this is to test your control solution (the control solution that comes with your meter has a known amount of glucose). Then compare the number on your control solution to what your meter reads. If the meter is accurate, the numbers should be the same.

Collected Tips

- I use the OneTouch Ultra meter these days and test the blood on my forearm. It's a whole lot less sensitive than the fingers.

  –Rollie Berry, age 18

- I use the InDuo. It's a OneTouch Ultra meter with a little blood test insulin-injection machine all in one (the Novo Nordisk insulin delivery system). There is a cartridge with insulin, and you screw on a pen needle and inject. It's neat. *–Drew Huver, age 7*
- I like the Dex meter because the strips are included in the meter. It's one less thing to forget. *–Jessica Stogsdill, age 18*
- When I was little, I tested one hand one day, one hand the next day. Now with my FreeStyle, I test the pinky side of the palm of my hand, between my wrist and the big line. *–Mo Lopez, age 10*
- To keep your fingers from getting overused, test your pinky before breakfast, ring finger before lunch, middle finger before dinner, and pointer finger before bed. Then use your right hand on even numbered dates and your left hand on odd dates. *–Childrenwithdiabetes.com chat room kid*
- Keep your monitor in the plastic case when you test, so it doesn't move around when you put your finger against the strip. I use the Ultra One. *–Evan McMillin, age 10*
- Test your blood sugar a lot even if you feel fine, just to stay in control. *–Renee Garcia, age 16*
- I use the OneTouch Ultra. My mom can test the top of my arm or do a finger prick. *–Anela Okamoto, age 3*
- Check your sugar a lot and pay attention to how you feel. *–Elizabeth Keylon, age 15*
- Test whenever you feel like something is not right. *–Jill Shatkus, age 16*
- Always test before going to bed. *–Michael Stack, age 17*

Finger prick testing is more accurate than arm pricks when your blood sugar is falling rapidly or if you are very low.

Pumps and meters that think

Bo: I was riding my bike across campus the other day when I met Mary Costello. We started talking about new stuff and our pumps when Mary said, "I'll bet I'm higher tech than you are."

I replied, "No! You have the Paradigm Link upgrade?"

"Yes!"

"Darn, I want one!"

Mary pulls out her advanced MiniMed meter that talks to her pump and showed me what it could do. Wow!

Mary: The Paradigm Link and Delta Cozmo pumps communicate to a meter. They allow you to input your own personal bolus ratios, basal rates, and point drop per unit rates (these rates can be different throughout the day). The pump analyzes your numbers along with your meter readings (blood sugar) and the amount of carbs you're eating—then suggests an insulin dose for covering highs and for covering food. It only takes a second. How cool is that? These pumps help you think.

The Paradigm 512 also allows you to set temporary basal rates, either as a percentage of your total basal or as a totally different basal value. Since I use various basal rates throughout the day, the percentage function is great for me.

- Upgrade: I upgraded through a Pathways program online at www.minimed.com. The upgrade costs $500.00 if you already have a Paradigm 511. Watch for special deals—I upgraded for $300.00. *–Mary Costello, age 21*

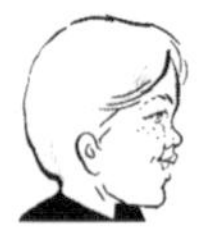

The new pumps allow for more precise doses, 0.05 unit increments instead of 0.1 increments—great for little kids!

The GlucoWatch

Jake Gershenson, 7, loves his amazing GlucoWatch. When he is not wearing it, he tests 8 to 10 times a day. When he wears his GlucoWatch, he just tests once every 12 hours. (The Gluco Watch needs to be calibrated once every 12 hours with a drop of blood.)

Jake's mom and dad say the GlucoWatch is a terrific tool for setting basal rates for the pump. For example, when Jake goes into a growth spurt, he puts on his GlucoWatch and sees his numbers every 20 minutes. Then he adjusts his basal rate accordingly.

The latest version of the GlucoWatch, G2 Biographer (made by Sankyo Pharma and Cygnus), gives a reading every 10 minutes and costs about $595 in the U.S.

Tip: I like my GlucoWatch. When we go on cruises and I go to the kids' club, I can just look at my watch and call my mom when I have a high glucose number, and she helps me figure out how much insulin to bolus. It doesn't work as well in hot weather, though.

–Jake Gershenson, age 7

Tip: I have a walkie-talkie, so when I am busy off playing, I can check in any time my GlucoWatch shows my sugars are straying high or low.

–Jake Gershenson, age 7

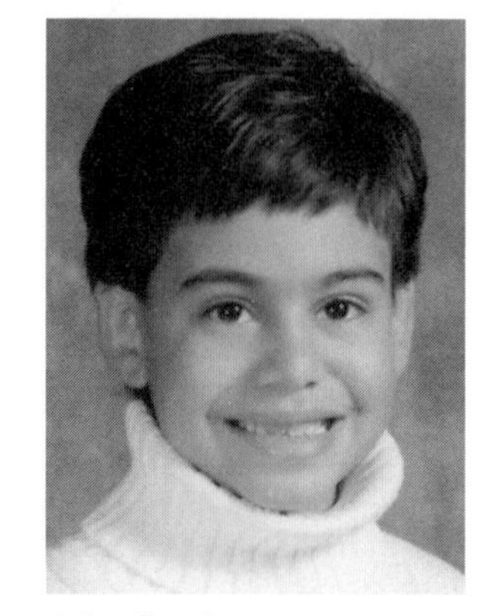

Jake Gershenson

Injection Devices

Spike: You can take your injections just about anywhere. Your thighs, arms, stomach, and the top round part of your hip are all good places. My parents used to give me my shots in my arms or legs. When I took over, I gave almost all of them in my hip (the very top of my butt). I let my girlfriend give me shots in my arms sometimes. It's important to switch injection sites to prevent one place from getting too sore, so I always gave my R shot in my left hip and my U shot in my right. If I were sore, I would inject in my legs. I tried my stomach but didn't really like it. Neither did Bo—he thinks it is because we are so "buff." I'm not so sure. . . .

My dad didn't like needles, which is not a great match for a kid with diabetes, so he would use an Inject-Ease to give me my shots. The Inject-Ease injects the needle so you don't need to do it manually. It also hides the needle, so you don't see it being injected. This would allow me not to be scared of getting my shot and would allow my dad not to be scared to give me my shot.

Since I was diagnosed when I was really little (at the age of 2), my parents tried to make the times I did my blood sugars seem fun. They would dance around and sing,

"It's finger time, it's finger time," and make testing seem like it was a joyous event.

- Emla Cream numbs the skin.

–Brittany Rausch, age 15

- You can inject through your clothes—I did when dressed formally, like for the prom. Just don't shoot through your belt . . . it bends the needle. Spike usually shot through his pants leg when on an airplane. *–Bo*

Bo: Since Derrick Crowe is pretty much our Gadget Kid, I was excited when I finally got to recommend something to *him.* Last year Derrick was talking to me on the phone about wanting to give himself a shot. I told him that when Spike injects, he just uses a syringe, but that I use a neat little device called an Inject-Ease. You drop the syringe into the rocket-ship-looking Inject-Ease and press a button. The device sends the needle into you fast. Then you push the plunger down to deliver the insulin. Derrick called a few days later. He got an Inject-Ease and has given himself his first shot!

Tip: When I was little, I used an Inject-Ease to give myself shots. It made it a lot easier. *–Elizabeth Keylon, age 15*

The Insulin Pen

Rollie: I carry a Humalog Pen in my pocket with several needle tips. It's more convenient than vials and syringes and doesn't need refrigeration once it's opened. Once the tip is on the pen, you just dial the dose and inject. One of the nice features about the pen is that you can tell how much insulin you have drawn up by the number and by the clicks. For example, if you are using your pen in a poorly-lighted place, like when you're camping, when you dial in your dose, the clicks tell you how much insulin you have drawn up.

–Rollie Berry, age 18

Tip: I like the pen because my mom doesn't have to help me with it. It makes me more independent. When I need insulin, I can just take out my pen and inject anywhere and nobody notices. I can just use my pen wherever I am.

–Megan Weitzman, age 10

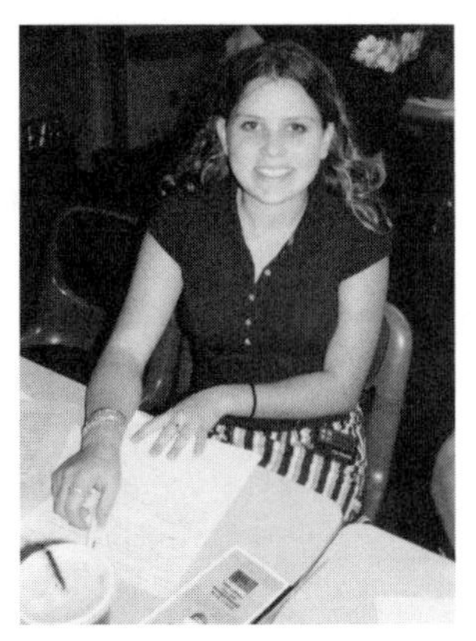

Brittany Rausch

Taking Care of Your Insulin

Kids always ask about how insulin that comes in bottles is made. The insulin we inject or pump is made in labs. The process is very high-tech. Scientists insert the human genetic code for insulin into bacteria or yeast, causing them to produce human insulin. They dilute it in liquid, package it in bottles, and we buy it from the pharmacy.

Insulin is a delicate protein that breaks down over time or in high temperatures (above 86°F) or freezing temperatures (below 32°F). It's the insulin we inject or pump that keeps our blood sugars down and keeps us healthy. Therefore, to take care of our bodies and manage our diabetes, we have to take care of our insulin.

- Never use insulin that doesn't look right. Humalog, Novolog, Regular, and Lantus (glargine) should look clear. NPH, Lente, and Ultra Lente should look cloudy. If you see particles floating around in your insulin, throw it out.
- Insulin can go bad. If you start to get high sugars a month or so into opening your bottle of insulin, try using a new bottle. But beware, new insulin can be much more potent than stuff that's a month old.
- Keep your insulin cool. Heat can alter insulin, causing long-lasting insulin to work like short-acting insulin, resulting in a very low blood sugar episode.

Tip: Throw away opened insulin after 30 days.
–Evan McMillin, age 10

Tip: Pump insulin gets old, too. If you are high all the time and you can't figure out why, maybe it's because your insulin is old. *–Mo Lopez, age 10*

Tip: If you leave your insulin in a hot car, throw it away and get a new bottle—better to waste a bottle of insulin than

Lantus Insulin

Lantus (glargine) is a new long-lasting (24-hour) insulin. Lantus is like the insulin the human body makes, and it gives your body a low level of insulin for twenty-four hours with no peaks. (Novo Nordisk will market a similar long-lasting insulin soon.)

Rollie: I started using Lantus insulin 2 months ago. It is really, really good. It's one step below using the pump. I take my Lantus at dinner because my dinner is usually consistent time-wise. I always have to take Humalog anyway, so it jogs my memory to take the Lantus. My doctor recommended Lantus at breakfast, but I like to have the option of sleeping in, so breakfast wasn't at a consistent time for me.

Lantus gives me a lot more flexibility with my meal times. In addition to the one Lantus shot a day, I take Humalog at every meal and large snack. I can do this any time of day. I can also skip meals and just not take a shot of Humalog.

to risk the high blood sugars damaged insulin can cause. *–Blair Ryan, age 16*

Tip: New insulin seems to have a little kick. Be prepared for a quicker reaction. *–Evan McMillian, age 10*

Tip: If you have a fever, the blood flow to your skin will be increased, and absorption of insulin will be quicker. *–Clare Rosenfeld, age 16*

Tip: Never share your insulin. Just to be on the safe side, you should only use your own insulin—insulin that you take care of yourself. *–Valerie Kintz, age 15*

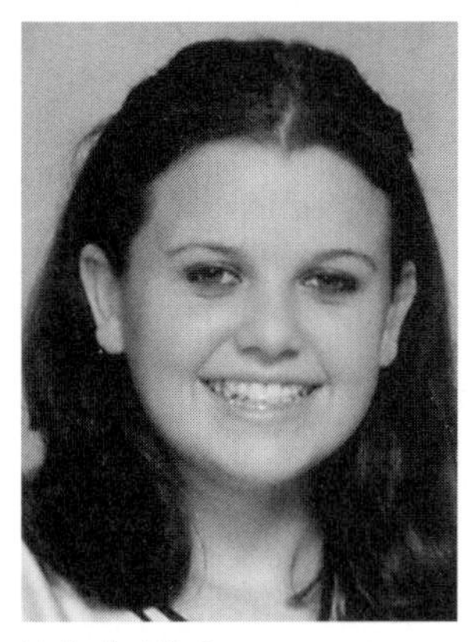

Valerie Kintz

Tip: I like these neat insulin holders (Insulin Vial Protectors, made by InSure) because they are good protection, and they feel squishy. We found them at Sav-On (drugstore). They cost about five dollars. When you travel or backpack, pop your insulin vials into padded holders. *–The Gadget Kid, Derrick Crowe, age 8*

Novolog insulin

Mary Costello: Novolog is a fast-acting insulin that works like Humalog. When I began getting little red marks at my pump site where the cannula was inserted, "pump bumps," I switched from Humalog to Novolog insulin. I am able to leave my set in for longer now, at least three days, and have no irritation with Novolog.

Kits and packs

We carry our diabetes supplies in Medicool's Dia-Paks. They have handy compartments for holding everything. We keep a granola bar in our kits, too.

Tip: Have two of everything. Keep a back-up kit at home in case you lose your main kit. *–Ryan Martz, age 20*

Tip: Fanny packs for my diabetes supplies are fun. I have several different colors and styles. They are big enough to hold my monitor and small snacks, but also small enough that they don't get in my way when I wear them. I take one with me whenever I am away from home.
–Kelly Hrubeniuk, age 10

Cooler

Bo: Spike and I have hauled coolers around for 15 years. We were the first kids at our elementary school to take their lunches to school in a cooler. Now all the kids do it! Our friends and families associate us with our coolers. They always know they can find snacks, quick sugar (glucose tabs or candy), directions on what to do if we are low (*Symptoms* taped into the top of the cooler), and our test kits in our coolers.

On vacation or when traveling with a team, we toss our glucagon kits in our coolers, and Voila! Everything is in one easy-to-find place. You might prefer to carry all your supplies in a soft cooler or a backpack. If you carry the same thing all the time, you and your friends will know at a quick glance if you have everything you need to head out on a road trip or go to the beach.

Spike: Our coolers were two of the most important things we had growing up. Bo's was red, mine was blue. We took our coolers absolutely everywhere, and we made sure they were fully packed every day with Gatorade, a tube of Cake Mate frosting for serious lows, granola bars, crackers, beef jerky, and caramels. We could go wherever we wanted to go and do whatever we wanted to do as long as we had our coolers.

- Keep a packed cooler in every car and one at school under your teacher's desk.
- Keep the cooler you carry to school packed and by the front door, so you don't forget it when you leave the house.
- Check your cooler's contents every day. Have Mom or Dad double-check it.
- Tape a copy of *Symptoms* (page 250) into the top of your cooler.

Tip: I take my cooler everywhere. *–Evan McMillin, age 10*

Medical ID

We wear Medical Alert ID necklaces. Some kids just won't wear a medical alert bracelet or necklace. There is a solution.

Rollie Berry told us about a website (www.medicassist. com) where you can get a watch online with the medical alert insignia on the face. When you purchase the watch, you can have whatever you want inscribed on the back. For example: I have diabetes. Or you can go to www.mediclidwatch.com and get a watch with a red insignia on the face and Diabetes written across the center of the face of the watch.

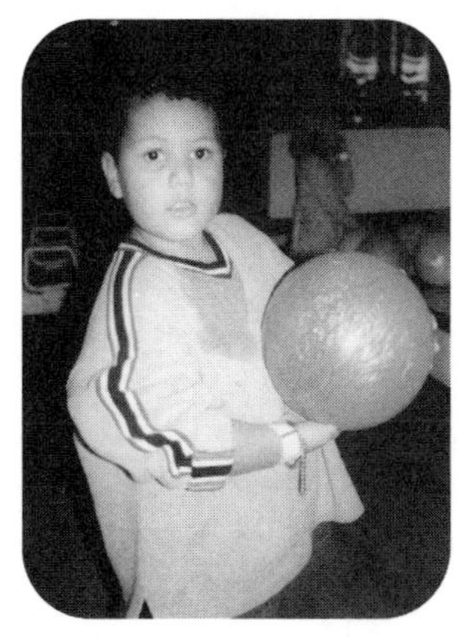

Trey Darensbourg

Tip: Always wear your Medical Alert ID bracelet.
–Trey Darensbourg, age 4 and Katie Tucker, age 13

Tip: I like my diabetes bracelet. I wouldn't like to sleep with a necklace.
–Laura Valine, age 5

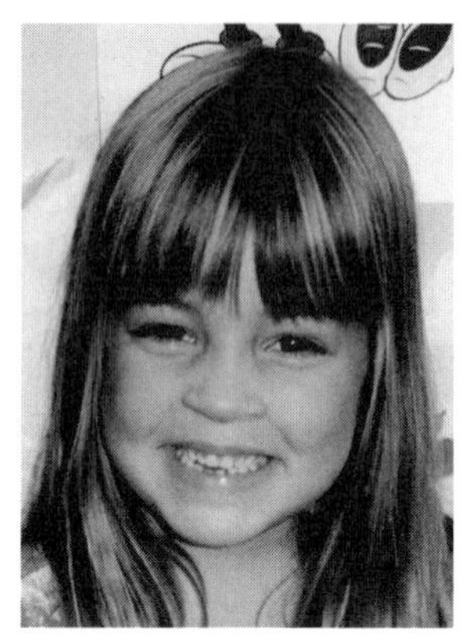
Laura Valine

Mary Costello has discovered a medical ID jewelry site. There are some awesome and beautiful medical ID bracelets, watches, and necklaces at www.laurenshope.com. The company was started because a girl with type 1 diabetes wouldn't wear a medical ID until her neighbor made these cute ones. I receive compliments on my bracelet all the time and people have no idea I wear it for medical purposes.

Tip: You can find awesome medic alert jewelry at www.laurenshope.com. It's so good it was in *People* Magazine. Halle Berry had some good things to say about them too.
–Mary Costello, age 21

You can also keep a Medical Alert Card in your wallet with more information. We write our parents' and doctors' phone numbers down on a little piece of paper and slip it into our wallets, next to our ID cards. No one has ever had to call these numbers, but it's nice to have them, just in case.

Syringes (and the fine art of collecting them)

Spike: I used to put my used needles into empty two-liter soda bottles. Once Bo got diabetes and the number of used needles doubled, we were filling bottles with syringes faster than we could drink all the soda. We had to upgrade. We started filling jumbo 5-gallon Sparklett's water bottles with syringes. It's cool to watch your bottle fill up. It was also a relief to quit having to drink all that diet soda.

It took a long time to fill our first 5-gallon bottle, but as we started taking more and more daily shots, our bottles filled up faster and faster. Now we have a collection of dozens of bottles stacked in our barn. When I travel I save all my used syringes (I put them in my soda bottles, just like I used to) and add them to the collection in the barn. Actually, it's kind of a pain to wrangle them out of the soda bottles, to put them in the Sparklett's bottles, so I usually let Mom do it.

Storing all our syringes almost makes injecting fun. I was actually excited when I went from 5 shots a day to 6 shots a day, because then I was able to fill a whole bottle on my own in less than a year.

- Be sure you take the needle off the syringe before you take the syringe to your kindergarten class for show and tell.
- Store your used syringes in those great big plastic water bottles.
- Try both BC regular and short needles. Different people find different length needles comfortable. I have always used the regular needle. Spike prefers the short.

–Bo

Tip: Instead of using the sharps container, get a Safe Clip. It cuts off the needle from the syringe and you can throw that puppy in the trash. *–Andrew Simecka, age 8*

Tip: Never share your syringes. *–Mo Lopez, age 10*

The Gadget Kid Says: Try New Things

Always be open to try something new, whether it is the pen, a new testing device, a Hemoglobin A1C testing system, or one of many new pump devices. You never know what's going to work best for you and keep you feeling good.

–Derrick Crowe, age 8

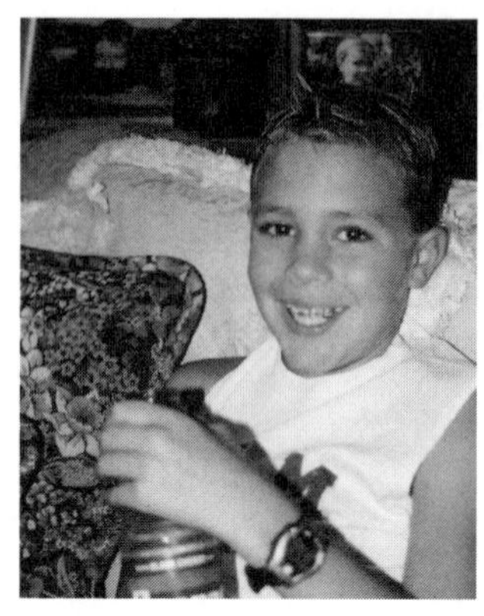

Derrick Crowe

CHAPTER SEVEN

The Adventures of Going on the Pump with Spike and Bo

Acknowledgments

Bo: Everybody we talk to who is taking three or more insulin injections a day is thinking about going on the pump. Spike and I hope our pump journal will help you make *your* decision. We were perfectly happy injecting insulin for the past 15 years, and now that we are on the pump, we absolutely love it.

We owe a debt of gratitude to many people for helping us become *pumpers*. We have to say a huge "Thanks" to Jackie Teichmann at the PADRE Foundation for her enormous energy, for all she does for kids, for setting everything up for us, and for suggesting we keep a journal. Thank you, Doctor Jody Krantz, endocrinologist, for taking good care of us, for contributing your wisdom to the pump journal, and for making it a better tool for kids and their families. Dr. Krantz is always available, which we all greatly appreciate. Our Certified Diabetes Educator, Debbie Warner, continues to do an outstanding job of educating us and all the other kids at Children's Hospital of Orange County (CHOC) about our pumps. Debbie is an incredible teacher; she is logical, patient, and gives freely of her vast knowledge and experience. Debbie is always ready to answer our questions; she even called us on Christmas Day!

We would like to thank Bobby Schwarz, our MiniMed sales rep, who was there the day we went on the insulin pump, enthusiastically cheering us on. Bryan, Christine, Ryan, and Tricia, the staff at PADRE, always make all the kids feel welcome there, even Spike and me. And then there are A.J. and Valerie, PADRE kids. They were there on day one, offering their support and laughing at our attempts at carb counting. Thanks to Mark Daniels, MD, pediatric endocrinologist, and Joan Cervisi, CPNP, CDE, at CHOC, for generously giving your time to review the manuscript. We appreciate our friend Lyra Halprin Jackson's valuable comments, too. A special thanks to our aunt, Gebo Berger, editor extraordinaire, for the hours you spent editing and for your support for this project. We would also like to thank Vanessa Svoboda for her enthusiastic support. And finally, thanks to the family—Jenny, Mary, Dad, and especially Mom—for being part of the pump team.

Introduction

Spike: While collecting the tips for this book, we met all kinds of kids with diabetes. After getting a good tip or hearing a particularly funny story about diabetes, we always tried to share our own tips with these kids. The one thing about which we really couldn't share any tips of our own was pumping. Well, that's not altogether true—we did both wear a pump with saline solution for a weekend with the PADRE gang—but that doesn't really count. After hearing so many good stories about the pump, we knew that sooner or later we would have to try pumping for real.

The Adventure of Beginning

Spike: We both went on the pump on the same day, right before Christmas. (Our mom tried to convince us that insertion sets and reservoirs were our Christmas presents.) We are very happy that we did. We've always had good control, but now it is even easier for us to do what we want to do, when we want to do it, and still have good numbers.

Sure, pumps take a little getting used to, but they really do make diabetes an even smaller part of our lives. I think about diabetes even less now than I used to. I don't have to—my pump thinks for me. Well, kind of, anyway.

So, now we have tips of our very own to share about pumping. Next time someone tells me about how she gets through swim practice on the pump (by just taking it off and taking quick breaks to test and bolus every half-hour or so), I will be able to tell her how to make your pump look cool when you are wearing a suit and tie. I am not sure if this will be a very useful tip for her, but at least I will have a tip about pumping to share. Actually, when I have questions about pumping, I usually have to call Bo.

"Bo, you awake?"

"Yeah, but why are you calling me at 2 AM?"

"Umm, I can't get my pump to work."

"Did you just switch the battery?"

"Yeah, how did you guess . . . ?"

"You put the new battery in upside down again. Take it out, toss it, and put in the new battery. This time put it in right side up. Good night." <Click>.

30 seconds later. . . .

"WHAT???"

"Hey, sorry to call you back. You were right. Thanks, Bo!"

<Click>

"Bo? Bo, you there . . . ?"

Spike: He didn't start hanging up so abruptly until the seventh time I called him in the middle of the night, during finals, with the same question. I am now proud to announce that it has been a solid three weeks since I have put in a battery the wrong way.

Bo would like to mention that he has never, not even once, made this mistake. As he put it, "Dude, there is a picture right there showing how to do it. Why don't you just pay attention to how the old battery was put in when you take it out? Do you know the difference between positive and negative? I can't believe you went to Stanford." He says that last line a lot.

We kept a journal for the first month after going on the pump. It was a remarkably easy transition, and we recommend pumping to anyone who wants to keep even better control of blood sugars. And when you are reading the journal, don't worry, anything that is at all technical was written by Bo.

Making the decision to go on the pump

Bo: You know the saying, If it ain't broke, don't fix it? Well that's been my motto. Having diabetes for 14 years, I had become very comfortable with the way I took care of it.

All of these things contributed to our decision to become pumpers, and I was reassured to know that if I didn't like it, I could simply go off the pump. At any time I could inform my diabetes educator that I wanted to go back to my old way of injecting insulin, and she would help me make the adjustments. Going on the pump is not a one-way street.

A smooth transition

Bo: The doctors want you to keep track of everything you do for a few days before you start the pump. You should come to your pump appointment with detailed records of what you ate, what your blood sugars were, what insulin you took, any exercise you had, and anything else that could affect your blood sugars and insulin levels. Also, to make things run smoothly, you should talk to your doctor beforehand to figure out what his or her record-keeping preference is. For instance, some doctors prefer that you write in a logbook, while others have the capability to download information off your meter, either a regular meter or one of the new palm pilot-based meters.

In preparation for going on the pump, you will meet with a dietitian to make sure you understand carb counting, and you will have a basic physical. You'll meet with your diabetes support team to learn how to program and use your pump.

There is a whole new vocabulary that goes with insulin pumping. Don't worry, it's easy to learn, and when your certified diabetes educator (CDE) shows you the ins and outs of using your insulin pump, the vocabulary will make sense. So, before we take off on our journey, here are some terms you need to know:

Terms to know

Basal—Background insulin, delivered continuously throughout the day and night. This is the insulin your body makes for activities other than eating.

Temporary basal (temp basal) – Change in regular basal rate for a short length of time (up to 24 hours).

Bolus—Insulin delivered on demand (like when you eat). A bolus covers the carbohydrates you eat at a meal or snack. Boluses also correct for high blood sugars.

Correction bolus—Insulin delivered to correct high blood sugar.

Suspending the pump—Stopping the pump from delivering insulin.

Carbohydrates—Foods that raise blood sugar: starches, such as bread, pasta, rice, starchy vegetables like potatoes; fruits and fruit juices; milk and milk products; and foods with natural or added sugar.

Rapid carbohydrates—Foods that raise blood sugars quickly: sugar, juice, candy, Cake Mate gel, glucose gel and glucose tablets.

Carbs (CHOs)—Carbohydrates.

Infusion site—The place on your stomach, hip, or thigh, or under your arm where you insert the cannula under your skin.

Cannula—The part of the pump system that you inject into your skin. It's a tiny, soft plastic tube.

Insulin-to-carb ratio—Number of carbohydrates covered by 1 unit of insulin. (If you take 1 unit of insulin to cover 10 carbohydrates, the insulin-to-carb ratio is 1:10.)

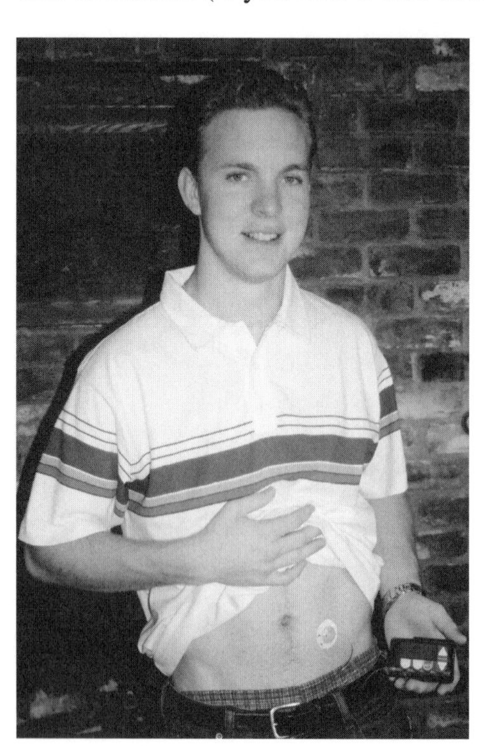

Bo shows off his pump at home.

Correction dose ratio—Number of points 1 unit of insulin lowers blood sugar. When you are experiencing high blood sugar, if 1 unit of insulin lowers your blood sugar 30 points, the correction dose ratio is 1:30).

Target range—The range of blood sugar levels where you want yours to be. For example 80–140 mg/dl.

HbA1C (Hemoglobin A1C)—Also called A1C. This is a blood test that shows your average blood glucose level over the past 60–90 days.

CDE—Certified Diabetes Educator

PADRE—Pediatric Adolescent Diabetes Research Education Foundation (padrefoundation.org)

CHOC—Children's Hospital Orange County

Kinds of Insulin

H—Humalog (lispro): fast-acting insulin
N—Novolog (aspart): fast-acting insulin
R—Regular: short-acting insulin
NPH—Neutral Protamine Hagedorn: long-acting insulin
Lantus—Glargine: 24-hour, long-acting insulin (new)
Lente—Long-acting insulin (rarely used)
Ultra Lente—Long-acting insulin

MONDAY DECEMBER 23

The Pump Story

Spike: We woke up at 4:30 AM and were on the road by 5:00. We were heading to CHOC, where we would officially become pumpers. There are plenty of places closer to Ojai where we could have plugged in for the first time, but we had a special deal with the people at CHOC. That day we were going to complete all the training, which is normally spread over several weeks, in a single day: pump trial, physical exam, lab workup, carb-counting class, and carb-counting test (and for me, another carb-counting review after I failed miserably the first time).

The night before going to CHOC, we tested, took our usual R at dinner, tested, and took NPH before bed. In the morning, we took our short-acting insulin, R, but no long-lasting insulin—no U, no NPH, no Lantus (not that we have ever used Lantus but we didn't take any of that either). The docs didn't want any long-lasting insulin still in our bodies when we started pumping.

I almost gave myself the morning NPH shot about three times. Once I even had the insulin drawn before I remembered that I wasn't supposed to shoot up. Old habits. . . . It's weird thinking that I may never (well, almost never) take any shots of insulin again. Not to say I'm going to miss them . . . well, except for collecting my used needles and filling those 5-gallon water bottles with them. Gonna have to get a new hobby.

Tip: Kids who are going to go on the pump are usually set up with fast-acting Humalog or Novolog by the diabetes team. The morning before their pump appointment, they take only Humalog or Novolog.

Tip: Going on the pump doesn't mean that you will never need an injection with a syringe again. Sometimes you may need to give insulin with a syringe if you go off the pump for a few days, if your pump malfunctions, or if you have high blood sugar and ketones.

We slept the whole way down while Mom drove. She wanted to come along to learn all about the pump, too. She said it was so she can help other moms with kids going on the pump. I think she came along to embarrass us. She must have taken 300 pictures during the course of the day. I'm glad she came though, and not just because I got to sleep on the three-hour drive there and the three-hour drive back. She also paid for breakfast.

We got to Orange County pretty early and went looking for McDonald's for breakfast. We couldn't find one and settled on Carl's Jr. We took regular insulin with our breakfast and headed over to CHOC for our first meeting of the day.

Our first official meeting was with Dr. Jody Krantz. We had a regular checkup, like we would with our own endocrinologist. Since it was our first time with an endocrinologist at CHOC, we had to fill out all the paperwork—the medical background, the family history (Mom got to do that—I guess it was a good idea to let her tag along). Then we went over our daily routine: How much we eat and when, how much we exercise, and how much insulin we take. Last, we went over the detailed records of food and insulin, etc. that we had been meticulously tracking for the past several days.

Why keep records for 3 days before your pump appointment?

Bo: It is important to keep detailed records for several days before you go on the pump. For Spike and me, it was only three days. You have to keep records of meals, insulin, and exercise, so that your doctor can figure out:

- What is your insulin sensitivity? My blood sugar drops 40 points for every 1 unit of insulin I take.
- What is your insulin-to-carb ratio? I take 1 unit of insulin for every 10 grams of carbohydrates I eat.
- What should your basal rates be? My basal rates are lower in the early morning.

Keep accurate records for a few days before you go in to start pumping, so your doctor can get you going in the right direction.

Figuring out your insulin needs

Spike: Right away Dr. Krantz suggested that I might be having hidden lows. She looked at how much insulin I was taking (about 70 units a day, which is kind of a lot for a trim, fit, muscular individual like me) and how much I was eating (not that much—I live away from home now and have to pay for everything myself), and concluded I was probably having a bunch of low blood sugars that I wasn't noticing. When she looked at my numbers, she had even more evidence, since my A1C was lower than it should be given my average blood sugars.

While Doc Krantz took our meters to download the past month of numbers, we went downstairs for a physical. The physical was pretty standard. She did a neat little test where you hold your hands flat together to make sure you do not have decreased joint mobility, listened to our hearts, and looked in our ears. (Apparently I have the waxiest ears she has ever seen. I figure it must be because I am so healthy, even my earwax-making cells are strong and robust. Bo thinks I am just gross.)

We also got our blood pressure checked and our height checked. (For the record, the height chart on the wall at CHOC is at least one inch off. I am 5'10"! I swear!) We also had our weight checked. (For the first time ever, Bo outweighed me—by half a pound—looks like I am going to have to start being nicer to the "little" guy.) We also had a finger prick for me and an arm prick for Bo for our A1Cs.

Figuring average blood sugar

After the blood sugar tests, Doc Krantz showed me the printout of my numbers and my A1C. My meter numbers showed an average of something like 187, which should correlate to an A1C of 8 to 9. My A1C was actually 7.4. That must mean I am having more low sugars than I know about, occurring in-between the times I was testing. Sometimes when I know I am low, I just eat and don't test, so that might explain some of it. In any case, it was a good reminder to see an endocrinologist four times a year. They are trained to figure this stuff out. It only took Doc Krantz 30 seconds to conclude that I was having hidden lows—something that never even crossed my mind.

It's especially important to see your endo when you are going through major lifestyle changes. I just graduated from college and moved out of the frat house into a place of my own a few months ago. I think that has contributed to my hidden lows and slightly higher A1C. My A1C was 7.1 in June; I bet with the pump I'll be there again in no time. An A1C-average glucose chart is on page 227.

Carb counting

Spike: Next we met with Newell McMurtry, our dietician, to take the dreaded carb-counting quiz. You have to be able to add up the carbs in different meals and figure out how many units of insulin they require. If you have a ham sandwich with two slices of bread and a glass of orange juice, how much should you bolus? The first questions were easier, because they told us how many carbs were in the food (15 grams of carbohydrate in each slice of bread, 15 g in 4 oz of OJ) and the ratio of insulin to carb we were using (1 unit of Humalog for every 15 grams of carbohydrate). So for our 45-gram carbohydrate meal, we would bolus 3 units. I aced that part. The next part, on the other hand. . . .

The next part gave lists of foods in a meal, and we had to say how many carbs were in each list. Let's just say that *Bo* passed this part. I screwed up on fruit salad, milk, OJ (and the answer to that one was on the first page), and pasta. If water had been on there, I would have gotten that wrong too. And the last question, something about an enchilada with tortillas, sauce, beans, rice, and a drink . . . forget about it.

For the next half hour or so, Newell walked me through carb counting from the top. By the end of it, I felt OK about the whole thing, but Newell suggested I take three books full of carb charts with me . . . everywhere I go . . . for the next six months . . . until I figure this thing out. Actually, I do have a decent handle on it. But the books are really helpful. My favorite is *The Doctor's Pocket Calorie, Fat & Carbohydrate Counter.* It gives the carbs for loads of foods and all the fast-food places to boot. I haven't eaten anything yet that I haven't been able to look up in that book. The same goes for *The Diabetes Carbohydrate and Fat Gram Guide* (ADA, new edition in 2004).

My family laughed at me for a while (Yeah, my sister was there too; Mary, Bo, and Mom all just cackled away at me) for not knowing that a potato has more carbs than a piece of celery. Once their fun ended, it was time to get down to the serious business. It was time to start pumping!

Pumping

Debbie Warner, our CDE, came in with some prop pumps for herself, Mary, and Mom. Bo and I got our own out. She taught me how to change the battery and reminded us that we have to put new ones in at least once a month. Bo had already put his battery in and was ready to get going.

Next we set the time and date—turns out I had my AM and PM reversed (more about that later). This little step can be pretty important, since you may be taking different basal rates at different times during the day. For instance, you may take more in the early morning and less in the afternoon. If your pump thinks it is 2:00 PM when it is really 2:00 AM, then your basal will be off, too. So, make sure you pay attention when the pump trainer tells you to make sure you set your time and date right.

After the initial setups were completed, we went through each step on our pumps.

- We learned different ways of giving boluses.
- We learned how to schedule different basal rates for different times of the day.
- We learned how to suspend activity (stop the pump) and how to restart it.
- We learned how to set temporary basal rates for when we are exercising or when we are sick or just need more or less insulin. (Girls often need temporary boluses during their periods, since their blood sugars can run higher.)
- We learned how to review our bolus history and more.

There are lots of little things to go over, but it is really quite simple. We are using MiniMed Paradigms and everything is pretty intuitive. You just hit the blue ACTivity button and pretty much follow the menus to what you want to do. (On the older pumps it's the Select button.) I had read over the instruction booklet the day before and was feeling a little intimidated. Walking through the steps with Debbie made everything clear and, as I said, using this model pump is pretty darn simple.

Next we learned how to prepare our tummies for the cannula—wipe stomach with IV prep and let it dry—and how to inject the cannula. We got to practice on a cute little fake tummy. Again, the steps are simple, but having someone show you once before you try it on yourself makes it a lot easier. Bo and I had actually practiced inserting the cannulas and wearing pumps around once before, at the PADRE Teen Retreat last summer at UCLA, but I was still grateful for the refresher course. We also went through the steps of filling the pump canister (reservoir) with H and connecting all the tubing.

Since we knew how to operate most of our pump features and how to get ourselves connected, the last step before we officially became pumpers was to set up the pump itself.

- First we input a basal rate. We both started with 1.0 units of Humalog per hour. Eventually we would both change the amount, but this seemed like a good number, based on the amount of insulin we had been injecting.

- Next we learned how to rewind the screw on the pump and to prime it, and how to fill the tubing with insulin so that once you connect the pump to your body, insulin will start pumping in.
- We also set our fixed prime for 0.5 units—more on this in a second.

It took about 10 units to fill my tube. Once the tube is full, you can see a little insulin dripping out the end of the needle. Once the pump is primed, it's ready to hook up to you. We put the insertion piece inside our Medtronic MiniMed Quick-Serters, peeled off the sticky paper, cocked our Quick-Serters, pulled off the blue safety caps, and were one step away from pumping.

Bo and I decided to inject the infusion site on the count of three. "One, two, three!" Debbie counted for us.

"Oh wait!" Bo shouted, "I touched the injection site!" Bo had touched the site he had just swabbed with IV prep and let dry. I had already injected though (it didn't hurt), so while he re-wiped and waited for it to dry again, I finished the last steps.

I pulled the Quick-Serter off and then pulled the needle out, leaving the soft plastic cannula behind. Then I smoothed out wrinkles in the sticky part of the cannula tape to get it to stick better and to make sure it wouldn't come off. (I think this looks kind of like a high-tech nicotine patch, so I call it "my patch.")

The last step was to activate the fixed prime. This sends insulin to the very tip of the tube. The plastic cannula in my body had no insulin in it (the needle did, but we had pulled the needle out), so we hit the fixed prime, and the insulin moved to the very end of the cannula. I was pumping!

Thirty seconds later, Bo was pumping too. He always said he was going to let me get on the pump first. He wanted me to be the guinea pig. Turns out I was, if only for 30 seconds.

Tip: Infusion sites, although primarily on the stomach, can also be in other locations as well—the top of the hip, in the hip pockets area, on the thigh, and at the edge of the breast or underarm.

How do you set the infusion site?

Bo: Everyone who is thinking about going on the pump wants to know what it is like to get hooked up to a pump. So, here it is, step by step.

- Fill a new reservoir with insulin. (I am a larger person, so I fill all 180 units on my Paradigm Pump.)
- Connect the reservoir to new tubing.
- Put the reservoir, which is now connected to tubing, into the pump.
- Prime it. Watch until some insulin drips out of the end of the tube.
- Inspect tubing to check for kinks and air bubbles. If air bubbles are present, I keep priming until all air bubbles are out.
- Answer all the questions on the pump screen. When the questions are answered, the pump says you are ready to go, and then you can insert your pump site.
- Now I stand up, relax, and look at my stomach to see where the little tiny red dot is from the last time. I make sure I choose a place on the other side of my stomach, 2 or 3 finger-widths away from my belly button, as well as 2-3 finger-widths away from where my last site was. I think about how my stomach feels, if I worked out hard, is one place sore? If so, I choose another site.
- Then I grab an IV prep swab, clean the area where I'm going to put the inserter (and use the rest of the swab to clean off the last spot of tape gum left on my stomach from the last site).
- Let it dry.

- I think about where the tubing will be aimed. If it's on the left side of my bellybutton I aim the tubing to the left, always towards the outside of my body, away from my bellybutton. If the site is really low, I aim the tubing up towards my bellybutton so it goes above my waistband. Otherwise you've got tubing looping under your waistband and back up again. I position it so the tubing aims towards my pants pocket.
- Put infusion set into inserter.
- Take off adhesive covering.
- Cock inserter.
- Take off blue cap.
- Put inserter up against stomach. (I make sure I'm relaxed.)
- Hit button, release it, and make sure it's in your stomach.
- I hold my finger on the blue piece of the inserter site and take off the inserter.
- Hold the white part (connected to the cannula) against your stomach and pull off the blue part, which is connected to the needle.
- Press down the tape to smooth out any little wrinkles.

If it hurts or feels uncomfortable, I lie down for a minute, and the discomfort usually subsides. It sounds like setting the infusion site takes a long time, but after you get used to it, the whole process takes about two minutes. Then I'm ready to go for three days.

Spike: My stomach felt a little funny for about 30 seconds after I injected that first time, but after that I could tell there was something on my skin, but it didn't hurt.

Tip: If it ever *really* hurts, it's not in the right spot. After an hour, if you're not comfortable, redo it. (Use new tubing, re-prime the pump, and reset it.)

Tip: Don't put the site in skin-folds or places you bend.

Tip: Some kids use Emla Cream to numb the skin or an over-the-counter cream called ELAMAX.

Tip: IV Prep helps the cannula tape stick so that activity (even underwater activity) doesn't cause it to peel off.

How does it feel to set the infusion site?

Bo: A concern everyone has is "How much does it hurt?" It "hurts" about as much as an injection, and for me an injection is usually painless. When I use the Quick Set, all I feel is the inserter slapping against my skin. I don't actually feel the needle go into my skin, I feel the pressure of the inserter.

Lunch: first time carb counting

Spike: We went out for lunch with AJ and Valerie, two PADRE kids. The sandwich place didn't have a Nutritional Information Guide, so AJ and Valerie counted our carbs for us. We decided my great big steak and cheese sandwich had 80 carbs. I tested and was 103, so I bolused 8 units for the 80 carbs. Two hours later, at 4:30 PM, I was 160, so we did a pretty good job counting carbs in our first meal.

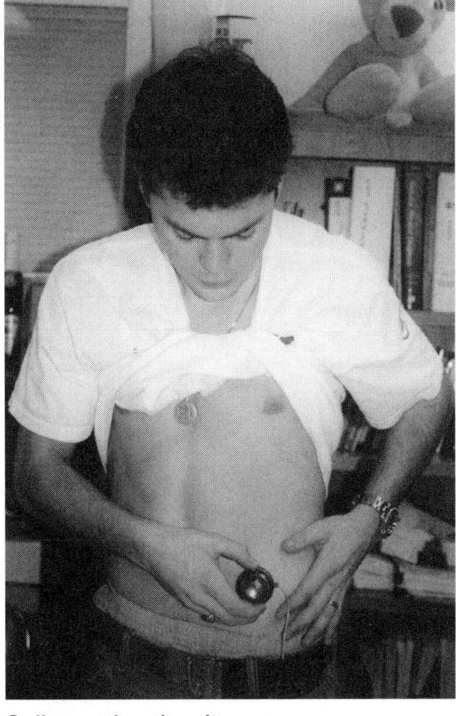

Spike setting the site.

After lunch we took some pictures with the PADRE gang and said good-bye. When we arrived home, it was time to test again. We were on a very tight testing schedule for the first 3 days to figure out what our basal rates should be.

DAY 1 MONDAY DECEMBER 23

Insulin pump start day

- **Blood glucose testing:** Test before every meal, two hours after every meal, at bedtime, at midnight, at 3:00 AM and 6:00 AM. Keep detailed records.
- **Meal planning:** Try to eat at home, keeping meals very simple and consistent. Try not to snack. This helps identify appropriate basal rates and bolus ratios. Plan for meals to be at the same time each day, with the same amount of carbs and same bolus. Choose easy-to-count carbs.
- **Physical exercise:** No intense physical activity, in order to establish accurate basal rates, insulin-to-carb ratio, and your correction factor.
- **Blood glucose target ranges:** Pre-meal, between-meal, and bedtime target range is 100–200. After the first week, the target range will be 80–160, two-hour post-meal target range, 100–180, and bedtime target range, 100–160. Tighter control will be achieved later (80–140). (For toddlers the starting target range is higher, 150–200. Consult with your CDE or physician.)

Spike: At 7:30 PM, my blood sugar was only 55, so I had 15 grams of carbohydrate (8 oz of Gatorade) and tested again in 15 minutes. At 7:45 I was at 88. I ate dinner then. Dinner was two small potatoes, chicken, salad, and 8 oz of milk. We counted that as 43 carbs, and I bolused 4.3 units. I tested about an hour after eating, at 9:00 PM and was right back to 55. I had 15 grams of carbohydrate and waited 15 minutes. At 9:15 I was 48! I had 30 carbs then (I was getting pretty sick of being so low) and was 66 at 9:30. I had 15 more grams of carbohydrate and at 9:45 I was 110. It seemed like my basal rate was probably a little high and that my bolus/carb ratio may be high too. But in order to really figure out what my ratio and basals should be, I needed not to change anything around until after I talked to Debbie. I decided to just be real vigilant and test a lot.

At midnight I was 101. Yeah! But at 1:30 AM I was 69, so I ate 15 carbs. I was 80 at 1:45 and decided to eat another 35 grams of carbohydrate and go to bed. I was tired—and sick of testing. Plus, my mom was going to wake me up again at 3:00 AM, so I figured I'd be all right. I woke at 3:00 and was 140. Yeah! But when my mom woke me up again at 7:15 AM (we were supposed to do it at 6:00 but we all slept through our alarms) I was back to 52. Boo! I had 15 grams of carbohydrate and at 7:30 I was 51. Twenty-one carbs and 15 minutes later I was 80. I had 12 more carbs and went to sleep (again leaving the job of waking me up in two hours to Mom). Looks like my basal rate was too high.

How does it feel wearing a pump?

Bo: I remember thinking that even if the insertion of the infusion site doesn't hurt, the infusion site stays in you the whole time—how is that going to feel? Don't worry. The needle that you use to set the infusion site is taken out as soon as you put the infusion site in. The only thing that stays in your body (or under your skin) is a little tube called a cannula. The cannula is made of a thin, soft, flexible type of plastic that makes it unnoticeable when you are wearing it.

How long does it take to quit noticing you are wearing a pump?

Bo: The first time I wore a pump I remember comparing it to wearing a Band-Aid. Does a Band-Aid hurt? No. How long does it take you to quit noticing it when you are wearing it? For me, I can notice a Band-Aid any time I want to. If I think about the fact that I am wearing one, I notice it, and the same is true of the pump. I find that in a matter of a minute or two I get used to the infusion site.

DAY 2 TUESDAY DECEMBER 24

Spike: I woke up at 11:00 AM and was 79. I had 60 grams of carbohydrate for breakfast (potatoes, toast, eggs, bacon, milk) and bolused 6 units of H. By 2:00 PM I was 80.

Changing the insulin-to-carb ratio

I called Debbie and told her about all my lows, and we lowered my basal to 0.9 between midnight and 6:00 AM and to 0.8 for the rest of the day. We also decided to change my insulin-to-carb ratio from 1:10 to 1:12.5 grams. That would mean I would be taking less insulin at each meal and have less insulin automatically pumped into me with my basal rate.

At 4:00 PM I hit the ESC button on my Paradigm to make sure I had made the changes to my basal rate properly. It said "Basal 1: 0.9U/H." That wasn't right. It should have been 0.8. I hit ESC again, then ACT to get to the menu, and checked my basal rates. They looked right: *1*) 12:00A 0.9U/H *2*) 6:00A 0.8U/H. I hit ESC 4 times to get back to the Status screen. It said I was getting 0.9U/H, even though it was 4:00 PM.

I scratched my head. I was about to give up and ask Bo for help when I checked the Status screen one more time. Sure enough, I had my AM's and PM's switched. I hit ACT, went down to Utilities and fixed the time. I was a little embarrassed, but I hadn't really done any harm. My basal rates were only 0.1 unit different from each other, and I had only been on the wrong rate for two hours. It was a good thing I checked though, because who knows when my basal rates might change by more?

I had one more low (69) that I treated with a mini juice box. Bryan and Christine had given us a whole case of these tiny little Juicy Juices that have exactly 15 grams of carbohydrate each. And they are tasty, too.

Write everything down the first three days you are on the pump

Bo: It is important to keep detailed records of insulin, food, and blood sugar levels for at least the first three days you are on the pump. This is the only way your doctor and CDE can help you fine-tune your basal rates and figure out your insulin-to-carb ratio (also called insulin sensitivity).

NO exercise

Bo: When my diabetes educator, Debbie, told me I couldn't exercise for the first three days on the pump I was frustrated. I am very active and love to exercise. I thought three days without exercise was going to drive me crazy. It all turned out OK, though. The reason they ask you not to exercise is to limit the variables to keep track of to just three: basal rates (baseline insulin), boluses (extra insulin taken when you eat), and carbohydrates.

The objective is to set your basal rates according to your body's natural rhythm. So if your doctor and diabetes educator keep track of your boluses, your meals, and your basal rates, they can figure out how your body works and then help you set different basal rates at different times of the day, so that your pump can act as your pancreas would.

In my case we did this by setting all the basal rates at 1.0 unit per hour. Then, through trial and error, testing before and after every meal, we determined my basal rates and insulin-to-carb ratio. My insulin-to-carb ratio is 1:10. This means I need to take 1 unit of insulin for every 10 carbs I eat.

Waking up at 3:00 AM, 6:00 AM, and 9:00 or 10:00 AM to test our blood sugar helped us determine our nighttime basal rates. I found that I was getting low a lot between 6:00 AM and 9:00 AM, so we lowered my early morning basal rates. In the beginning we set my insulin-to-carb ratio at 1:15. I got high after meals so we adjusted my insulin-to-carb rate down, settling on a 1:10 ratio to lower my post-meal blood sugar levels.

DAY 3 WEDNESDAY DECEMBER 25

Spike: The night went smoothly, and the next morning I woke up at 72. A little low, but not too shabby. That afternoon, though, I bottomed out. At 2:00 PM I was only 44 and ate up 50 carbs. By 2:25 I was 71, and I had 55 carbs for lunch. I bolused just 3.5 units since I was so low. I should have taken a little more because by 4:00 PM, I was 204. My first high sugar since going on the pump. I dialed in 2 units to correct for the high blood sugar and was 160 at 4:30. My lower basals and bolus/carb ratio helped me avoid any more lows that day. Hooray for Debbie!

Treating lows

Bo: When I was on injections, the only way for me to treat lows was to eat. But now, on the pump, I can both eat and lower my basal rate with a temporary basal to treat a low. For the first week or so, when I was in close contact with Debbie, I had to treat lows in a regimented way. I was to eat 15 grams of a fast-acting carbohydrate, then test in 15 minutes. If I was still low, I was to repeat the process: eat 15 grams of carbohydrate, then test in 15 minutes. If my numbers were OK, I was to eat another 15 grams of a longer-acting carb, and then take 1/2 the insulin I would normally take for the second serving of long-lasting carbs (page 222).

So, if I tested and was 60, then I drank 4 oz of orange juice (15 carbs). If I tested again 15 minutes later, and I was 100, then I would have 7 crackers (15 carbs). My insulin-to-carb ratio was 1:10, which meant I was supposed to have 1.0 unit of insulin for 10 grams of carbs. Since I was low, I only took 1/2 of my insulin-to-carb ratio (for the 15 carbs of crackers only), so I took 3/4 of 1 unit of insulin.

I find that when I am low at night, after I have already had dinner or my last nighttime snack, I might have a half serving of OJ and lower my basal rate from 1.0 to 0.5 for an hour, calculating that half a unit less of insulin would raise my blood sugar by about 20 points, and the half serving of OJ would raise it by another 20 points.

It's fun to see what you can do with the pump, but if you are going to try something new, make sure to run it by your CDE before trying it.

Tip: It takes insulin levels in your blood stream about 1 to 1 1/2 hours to kick in. Adjusting your basal insulin rate down may work for preventing lows, but it is too slow when your blood sugar is 70 or below.

Tip: If you test and are below 70, treat with carbs:15 fast carbs (such as 4 oz juice); wait 15 minutes; test; and follow with 15 grams medium carbs (such as crackers) (page 222).

First shower

Spike: The other exciting event of the day was my first shower. On vacation I try to shower at least twice a week, so waiting until Wednesday night wasn't really anything out of the ordinary. I was a little curious about how I'd do it with this pump thing, though.

I had a very hard time disconnecting the pump from my body. You just have to push in these little tabs and twist, but I felt like I was going to either break the little plastic thing or rip it out of my body. Neither of those seemed like a good idea, so I was very gentle with it. Finally I got it off. Seriously, I spent four minutes working at the thing. The shower was swell, and when I stepped out, I no longer smelled like someone who hasn't showered in almost 3 days. That was nice.

Reconnecting the pump to the insertion site was another nightmare for me. I was trying to push in the little clips and turn the thing gently. It just wouldn't work. Finally I twisted so hard, I was sure I was going to break something, when it actually twisted into place. I was back to being a bionic man—a pumper. I decided that it was so hard to take on and off, though, that I might just never shower again.

Oh yeah, Christmas was good too. I got some tools and a cheese board.

Detaching your pump

Bo: When I heard that MiniMed's new Paradigm Pump was water-resistant, I thought that was really cool; I wouldn't have to be careful around water. I remember thinking that I wouldn't wear the pump when I went surfing, and I wouldn't want to wear my pump wakeboarding in a lake because it might fall off and get lost like George's did (page 27). So for most water activities, I will simply detach my pump.

Tip: It's better to detach your pump and just let a little insulin drip out of the end of the tubing when showering, swimming, surfing, and during contact sports rather than setting your pump on the Suspend mode. When you suspend the pump, air can back up into the tubing.

I asked my CDE, Debbie, how hard it was to detach the pump. She said it was really easy, and it is. I would say that it is easier for me to detach my pump than it is to get out my cell phone and make a call. (And I would say it is awfully hard for me to figure out how to use my cell phone. . . .–*Spike*) To detach the pump, simply grab the infusion site, pinch the sides of the plastic infusion set, and twist it off.

Tip: Never sit in a hot tub without detaching your pump. Insulin is very sensitive to heat. Hot water will ruin your insulin. The same goes for taking hot baths.

Tip: **Never bolus before you get into a hot tub.** The insulin absorption rate soars in hot water, and you could crash.

Tip: The warranty on pumps covers everything technical that can go wrong with a pump. But if you lose it, it's gone.

Tip: Check with your homeowner's insurance. You may be able to add your pump, Palm Pilot, and meter to your policy.

Suspending your pump

Spike: You are only supposed to suspend the pump when you take it off for an extended length of time, say half a day or more. Someone could also suspend it for you if you were super low and didn't want any insulin going into your body. So it is good to know how to do it. On our pump, all you have to do is hit

ACT, then arrow down once to Suspend and hit ACT twice. After you hit ACT the first time, you just follow the instructions on the screen. To reactivate the pump, hit ACT twice. I'm telling you, these Paradigms are easy. My mom can use it! (I think it is more appropriate to say that these Paradigms are so easy even Spike can use it! –*Bo*)

Tip: Two good reasons for just letting a little insulin drip out when your pump is detached instead of suspending your pump: *1*) it's easy to forget to resume pumping when it's suspended. *2*) air bubbles can develop in the tubing when the pump is suspended.

DAY 4 THURSDAY DECEMBER 26

Changing Basals

Spike: I talked to Debbie about my afternoon low the day before. We decided to change my basals around a little bit again. She called it fine-tuning. We set it like this:

1. 12:00A 0.9U/H
2. 6:00A 0.8U/H
3. 2:00 P 0.7U/H
4. 9:00 P 0.8U/H

Debbie looked over my 3 days of detailed numbers including basals, boluses, carbohydrate intake, and blood sugars and came up with this regimen. You can see that it is really important to take detailed records your first few days and to talk with your pump specialists, so they can help figure this stuff out for you.

Fine-tuning your basal rates

Bo: How often should you reset your basal rate? Reset your basal when you start seeing your blood sugar drifting up or running too low, like Spike's. For example: If your target range is 80–140 and you're seeing 160s with an occasional 180 or 200 sugar, it's time to reset your basal. Reset your basal just like you did in the beginning.

This takes some work: extra testing; eating three simple, easy-to-count carbohydrate meals that day; and cutting out all extra variables like exercise. You'll need help from your CDE or your physician.

Nighttime basal rate

Bo: Check your nighttime basal rate every few weeks. You want to have good, level sugars at night. That means waking up at 3:00 AM and testing your blood sugar every once in a while. If you start seeing high or low blood sugars (sugars out of your target range) when you wake up in the morning, it is time to check your nighttime basal rate.

Tip: Make sure you have your AM and PM basal rates on your pump set with AM meaning morning and PM meaning evening. (Especially you, Spike.)

Temporary basal rate

Bo: When I was taking injections, if I felt like I was getting low or dropping, the only thing I could do to bring my blood sugar up to the appropriate level was to eat. I can remember countless times over the years when I would eat a large dinner and be really full afterwards, only to test an hour later and find out that I was low. It's true that I love to eat, but when I am that full, trying to drink 8 ounces of orange juice or eat a granola bar is a pain in the butt.

With the pump I find that I can lower my basal dose, which slows down the flow of insulin. This works well during the day when I can re-activate my basal dose to its original setting an hour or two later. At night when I see my numbers coming down or anticipate a low due to exercise, I simply set a temporary basal rate and lower my temporary basal rate for the next hour or so. You can even set the temporary basal rate to 0.0 or 0.1 units for as long as needed. When I set my temporary basal rate to 0.0, it automatically goes back to my regular basal rate after the desired time. (Suspending your pump is not recommended because you may forget to re-activate it, and while the pump is suspended, the tubing sometimes gets air bubbles.)

Changing the site

Spike: Thursday was our third day of being on the pump, which meant it was time to switch sites. It's awfully easy to take your patch off. **You don't even have to suspend your pump when you pull it off.** Bo pulled his pump out fast and kept making fun of me for how slowly I peeled the tape off my stomach. One little edge had already started to peel (one more reason not to take a shower?), so I just grabbed it and slowly pulled up. Little by little the patch came up. I thought it would hurt, but luckily I don't have a lot of stomach hair . . . yet. It didn't even hurt as much as taking a Band-Aid off. I also thought that when the actual cannula came out, it might hurt, but as I watched the little piece of plastic tubing come out of my stomach (a little bent for some reason), I didn't feel a thing. I was pretty relieved that it didn't hurt.

There was a little circle of sticky goo left where the edge of the patch had been and a tiny little red dot where the cannula had been. Debbie said we could just wash it with soap and water or wipe it with alcohol and the goo would come off, but I kind of liked it. It looks like a little bull's-eye. Anyway, I figured that if I ever showered again, it would come off then.

After that I filled the reservoir with insulin, threw away the special little blue cap/needle that comes with it, connected it to my tubing, rewound my pump, screwed in the reservoir, set up the Quick-Serter, and injected. Didn't hurt a bit. I told Bo the reason it didn't hurt on me was because I had the strongest stomach in the world. He said it probably hurt less on fat than muscle.

Tip: You should not change your pump site right before you go to bed, because if it malfunctions, you won't know it until you wake up 8 hours later (or for Bo on the weekends, 15 hours later). By that time you could be getting pretty sick from ketones.

Tip: If you do change your site before bedtime, double-check your blood sugar later in the night to make sure your pump is working!

Tip: Always check your blood sugar 2–3 hours after changing your pump site to make sure your pump is working.

Adding variables: exercise (cutting wood)

Bo: Since we weren't supposed to exercise for the first three days on the pump, on the morning of the fourth day I woke up early, got out my chain saw, and set out to cut about four cords of wood (four large truck beds filled to the brim with logs).

This was a lot of exercise, and the first day I ate a huge breakfast of bacon and eggs, toast, and milk (which I bolused for). During the entire day of cutting wood, I drank three 32-oz Gatorades and ate two granola bars and two Snickers bars (no bolus, lots of testing). Lunch consisted of a burger, fries, and a diet Coke (I bolused for lunch). My point being that I ate a lot of food to account for all the energy I was expending.

Even after eating all of this food and drinking Gatorade and orange juice at the first feeling of having low blood sugar, I never managed to get my blood sugar above 80, and it got as low as 55. This meant I had to stop using the chainsaw frequently, because it would have been dangerous for me to use it when my blood sugar was low.

The next day I got up early to cut more wood. I didn't feel like eating so much, so I decided to try something new. Instead of consuming lots more carbohydrates than usual, I just turned on my temporary basal and lowered it from 1.0 unit per hour to 0.5 units per hour. This helped a lot.

From that first experience of exercising on the pump, I learned that the pump gives you the freedom to change the amount of insulin you are getting with the push of a button. When I was on injections once I took my long-acting insulin, it was set in stone. I would have 14 units of Ultra Lente or NPH acting in my body. The only way to avoid or treat lows was to eat. But now on the pump, I can lower my basal rate to avoid low blood sugars later on, after exercise. This is quite a lifestyle change. Sometimes it's hard to believe that I don't have to constantly anticipate when the NPH is going to kick in . . . because on the pump, there is no NPH.

Tip: You always need to have some insulin on board. If you disconnect from your pump for swimming or surfing, make sure you reconnect every two hours and bolus a little insulin. You always want some short-acting insulin in your system.

Tip: Sometimes following heavy exercise some people have lows later . . . much later. For example, they exercise during the day and go low that night. You can set a separate set of basals for exercise days. The pump allows you to have different basals for different days. For example, basal schedule 1 for regular days and basal schedule 2 for exercise days.

Goo

Spike: Today I finally figured out how to disconnect and reconnect the Paradigm to the insertion site. I felt so stupid for having had such a hard time. Anyway, I realized that the two clips aren't on the same side of the little plug-in deal. That helped. I also learned that if you push the clips in a twisting motion and continue that twisting motion, the thing comes off very easily. I was stunned at how easily it came off this time. I was so excited that I clipped it back on (when you clip it on, you don't have to push in on the clips, you just line it up and twist) and repeated the steps about 5 times. On, off . . . on, off . . . on, off. I got really good.

I also noticed that the goo from my first patch didn't come off very well in the shower. I had to kind of scratch it and that left a bright red mark on my poor tummy. After the shower, I ran some IV prep over it as Debbie recommended, and it came right off. That Debbie, I tell you, she has all the answers.

Tip: Uni-solve is a solvent that takes the tape goo off.

Sleeping with your pump

Bo: The pump gives me more freedom than I ever could have imagined when I was taking injections. It used to be that the long-acting insulin I took the night before would dictate when my sugars would either start to fall or rise in the morning, thus dictating when I had to wake up. But working closely with my diabetes educator, we have programmed my pump with basal rates that fit my lifestyle. Now I can sleep in as late as I want.

On injections, when I woke up at 6:00 AM, my blood sugar was often on the low side. But if I woke up later, say at

10:00 AM, my liver would have secreted some sugar, so my blood sugars would be good. Also, sometimes when you sleep late, your NPH runs out, so when your liver kicks in the wake-up sugar, your blood sugar rises; if I slept in until noon, my sugars would be high.

With this in mind, we lowered my 6:00 AM basal rate to 0.8, kept my 10:00 AM the same at 0.9, and raised my noontime rate to 1.0. Now I can sleep as late as I want. I can even skip meals!

Pockets in your pajamas?

Bo: At first I thought I would need to start sleeping in shorts or pajamas with pockets to keep my pump in, but I have always liked to sleep in boxers, and I have found that boxers still work with the pump. The clip on the pump is strong enough to stay attached to my boxers. In the off chance that the clip slips off, the infusion site is stuck to my body so well that when the pump does tug on it, nothing happens and nothing hurts. It just feels like a Band-Aid being tugged on. The same goes if the pump falls out of my hand when I am standing up. There is just a tug, nothing else.

Tip: You can just lay your pump on the bed beside you or put it under your pillow. Experiment a little and you'll find out what works for you.

Tip: Some kids like to put their pump in a baby sock and pin it on their pajamas at mid-chest. If you don't sleep flat on your stomach, this works.

Tip: There have been reports of people who bolus in their sleep . . . kind of like sleepwalking, they sleep-bolus. The remedy is to use the child lock function at night, then turn off the lock when you get up in the morning.

Air Bubble

Spike: While sitting in the car waiting for my mother to come out of the post office, I noticed something funny about my tubing. There was about a 2-inch part right in the middle that looked different from the rest. I thought it might just be the light, but when I held it up for a closer look I could tell that the section had an air bubble in it. My whole 43-inch tube holds about 10 units, so I figured two inches would be about 1/2 unit. Since my afternoon basal is set at 0.7 U/H, that would mean I'd get about half as much insulin as I'm supposed to for the hour when the bubble was getting pumped into me. That's not good.

Since the cannula isn't hooked into a vein or anything, there isn't any serious danger from having a tiny bit of air in the tube, but it could be enough to screw up my numbers. Having mastered the art of disconnecting the pump from the insertion site just the day before, I took action immediately. (I was so proud of myself for being able to disconnect without having to ask Bo for help.) I just disconnected and bolused 8 units while disconnected—so the insulin just dripped out the end.

I watched the little air bubble move down the tube. When it reached the end of the tubing, the dripping of insulin ceased until the whole bubble was out and insulin again pushed through. I reconnected after my pump beeped to indicate the bolus was finished and tested an hour later to make sure my pump was working.

Since my pump now thought I took those 8 units, my history would be a little skewed. I made a note of it in my logbook. Next time I fill a new reservoir I am going to be extra careful about tapping all the air out.

Tip: Any time you think your pump is not delivering insulin or working properly, trouble-shoot your pump. **Always**

test an hour after trouble-shooting or resetting your pump site to make sure your pump is delivering insulin.

DAY 7 SUNDAY DECEMBER 29

Trouble-shooting

Spike: I had two cheeseburgers for lunch (without the sauce). I was 97 when I sat down to eat and counted the two burgers as having about 60 total grams of carbohydrate (15 per bun, 2 buns per burger). With my insulin/carb ratio of 1:12.5, I bolused a total of 4.8 units. I figured it like this: 2 units per 25 carbs, so 4 units for the first 50 carbs. Then 10 carbs requires about 8/10 a unit of insulin, so I need a bolus of 4.8.

About 15 seconds after I had hit ACT to start the bolus, my pump beeped at me. It wasn't a nice beep, so of course I looked at the screen. It said, "Delivery stopped." I hit the ESC key to check my history. It said, "Last Bolus 2.6U." That meant I had only gotten 2.6 units instead of the 4.8 (4.8 – 2.6 is 2.2), so I still needed 2.2 units.

I checked my tubing and sure enough there was a tight little knot in it. I am not sure how it got there, but I loosened it and untied it by pulling the whole pump through the loop. Then I took another bolus of 2.2 units. There was no problem this time.

AJ said this kind of thing just happens sometimes, and usually it's just a kink. AJ and Valerie recommended disconnecting and reconnecting the pump from the infusion site if you can't find a kink.

Tip: You can always call the pump manufacturer's 24-hour help line if you can't figure something out. For MiniMed, the 24-hour pump help-line is 800-826-2099.

DAY 8 MONDAY DECEMBER 30

Racquetball

Bo: My first racquetball game since going on the pump was with Phil Schmit, someone I hadn't played since going away to college. Phil, a friend of my folks, is an old racquetball player with an amazing serve. Back when I was in high school and just starting to play racquetball, Phil took great pleasure in beating me (and had been gloating about it ever since). This time things were different. I annihilated him!

I've been playing a lot of racquetball at USC and have figured out what works for me. I test right before I play. If I am over 160, I bolus some insulin. If I am under 120, I drink some Gatorade. Before the game starts I go ahead and disconnect my pump, put it in my gym bag, and play without it. You can get hit by the ball—that's why I disconnect when I play.

After playing for about 45 minutes, I check my blood sugar to see where I am. I like to play with just 0.1 or 0.2 units of insulin in my system, so I have a little insulin working but I'm not running on empty. I check every 45 minutes during play. Once my blood sugar gets above 180, I take a correction bolus. If I test and I am under 120, I eat something.

Racquetball is an all-out sport. You use a lot of energy, sweat a lot, and need to stay hydrated throughout tournaments. I constantly sip Gatorade, no matter how many games I play.

DAY 9 TUESDAY DECEMBER 31

Dressing Up

Spike: On New Year's Eve, I had a dinner date with Vanessa and my best friend Andrew and his girlfriend. It being New Year's, I decided to get marginally dressed up. Luckily I got a new shirt-with-buttons for Christmas or I would have had to borrow something from Dad. That is never good.

Tucking in a shirt has always been hard for me, and now I had to deal with all this tubing. I think I figured out the trick. You want to be sure you have some extra tubing on the inside of your shirt so there is slack. If the tubing is pulled too tight, you will feel a little tug at your skin where the patch is stuck to you. So I gathered some slack, tucked it on the inside of my shirt, tucked my shirt into my pants, and put the leftover tubing into my pocket where my Paradigm was clipped. I looked sharp. Even Vanessa said so.

Tip: You can cut a slit in your pocket and run your tubing through it.

Beer

That night I had a few beers to bring in the New Year. They were light beers, so they only had about 6 carbs each. So the 24 carbs I drank, spread over about four hours, didn't have a real big effect on my blood sugar. In fact, when I tested back at home, I was 87. I hadn't bolused since dinner (Mm, prime rib) and was a little worried that the alcohol might cause me to crash in the middle of the night.

I decided to eat about 21 grams of carbohydrate (one king-sized chewy granola bar—you can get them in bulk at Costco). I also lowered my basal by setting a temporary basal. I went to bed at about 1:30 AM and figured I would be getting up at about 11:30, so I set the time for the temp basal at 10 hours. I had no idea how much insulin per hour to set, but I knew I wanted some, so I set it at 0.1U/H to be on the safe side. Turns out this was a little low.

Tip: Drink in moderation.

Tip: Two beers can cause you to have low blood sugar in the wee hours of the morning. When your liver is busy filtering alcohol, it does not release sugar into your bloodstream. This is important, because it's the sugar released into your bloodstream by your liver that your nighttime basals are meant to cover.

Tip: Be sure you eat some carbs, protein, and fat while drinking beer and before you go to bed.

Tip: Check your blood sugar before going to bed and again in the middle of the night.

DAY 10 WEDNESDAY JANUARY 1

First High Sugar

Spike: I woke up at about noon and tested. I was almost 300, my highest sugar yet. Looks like I shouldn't have turned my basal down so much. I took a correction bolus of 5 units and was 120 an hour later. Next time I drink beer at night, I will turn my temp basal down to about 0.5 instead (about 1/2 my normal basal rate) and see how that goes. If I am low, of course, I will eat; and if I am very low, I may turn the basal down lower. Waking up at 300 isn't a good thing, but it's not the end of the world either, since I can always correct the high sugar with a bolus.

Treating highs

Bo: For the first few days, I only treated highs when my blood sugar was 200 or above (my target level was 150). So if I was 170, I wouldn't take a correction bolus (a bolus you take just to correct your blood sugar when it is too high).

At 200, I would normally take 2 units to bring myself down to 120, but since my target range was 150 for my first few days on the pump, I would only take a correction bolus of 1.2 units.

DAY 11 THURSDAY JANUARY 2

Jogging

Spike: Vanessa finally convinced me to go running with her. I clipped my pump onto the inside of my waistband, tested (I was in my target zone), had a swig of Gatorade, and was ready to go. Vanessa is a good runner, but she slowed her pace a little, so I wouldn't die. Thank goodness! After about 2.2 miles, I had had enough and walked the rest. She ran ahead another mile before turning around. After she met up with me, we walked the rest of the way back together.

"How's the pump with running?" she asked.

This was my chance. If I could just tell her that it hurt terribly and that I was in agony, not only would I not have to go running anymore, but also she might run back to the house and come pick me up with a car!

"Actually," I started, "it doesn't hurt at all." Doh! I blew my perfect chance to get out of running. But the truth is, it really didn't hurt. I didn't even notice that it was there.

"Great!" she chirped, "Shall we make it three miles tomorrow? How about at say . . . 8:00 o'clock?"

Why didn't I just lie?

DAY 14 SUNDAY JANUARY 5

Changing the Site Again

Spike: I changed my infusion site today and had a bit of a problem. I inserted it and, before pulling the needle part out, I leaned down to pick up the Quick-Serter, which I had dropped on the floor. I think the needle must have been right in a muscle because it hurt pretty bad. I let out a little yelp and gingerly pulled the needle out. My poor tummy was sore for the next hour. There was a dull ache there. I considered pulling the whole thing out and switching back to the other side of my stomach for the next three days. After a while, though, it no longer bothered me.

From now on, I will not bend over with the needle in me. I will also be making more of an effort to avoid injecting anywhere near the muscle on my stomach. Looks like I am going to have to stop going to the gym, so I don't get too muscle-y. Hey, I guess that means I can't run with Vanessa anymore either. Dang.

Tip: Don't bend over before you remove the blue plastic inserter.

Tip: Don't insert in places you bend.

DAY 15 MONDAY JANUARY 6

Snowboarding, High Altitude, and Heavy Exercise

Bo: After wearing my pump for two weeks, I went to Whistler, Canada, for a five-day snowboarding trip. I learned very quickly (forewarned by my CDE) that I would need a lot less insulin at high elevations and even less during extreme exercise like snowboarding for six hours straight.

Besides the regular stuff, such as taking along lots of granola and candy bars in case I got low and having $20 in my pocket in case I needed to buy food, I learned that the easiest way to keep my blood sugar stable was to lower my basal rates for all hours of the day by about 20%. I did this by setting a new pattern. I also lowered my basal rates further when I knew I would be snowboarding. For this I would go into Temporary

Basal Rates and change it to about half of my normal basal rate. If I was going to be snowboarding for five hours, half an hour before I went on the slopes, I would change my basal rate to 50% lower, and I'd leave my basal rate lower for at least an hour after my exercise was done.

Tip: Be sure your tubing is all tucked in close to your body to keep it from getting snagged and to keep it warm. If the pump or tubing should freeze, you could be in for a problem.

Tip: Insulin doesn't work when it has been frozen, even after it thaws out.

Tip: The protocol for high altitude and the pump is to lower both your basal and bolus rates by 10% to 20% while at high altitude. This amount varies from person to person.

Tip: When you add exercise to high altitude, you may need to adjust your basal by lowering it according to how hard you exercise. (I also lowered my bolus by about 30%. When I would usually take 9 units of insulin to cover 90 carbs, I took only 6 units.)

Tip: Check and see what adjustments work for you. The rate of adjustment can vary from a 10% decrease all the way up to a 75% decrease if you are really exercising hard all day.

Tip: The better physical shape you are in, the less you have to adjust your basals.

Tip: Some people have high blood sugars at high altitude, so frequent testing is important to help you figure out what works for you.

DAY 20 SATURDAY JANUARY 11

Blue Safety Cap

Spike: The time had come again for changing the insertion site. It is amazing to me how quickly three days come and go. I am pretty used to using the Quick-Serter to inject myself but am still a little jumpy around the thing. (You would think after taking up to 7 shots a day for 15 years I wouldn't be such a baby.) Anyway, I set everything up and held the Quick-Serter up to my stomach (back to the left side again). I took a few deep breaths and hit the buttons on the sides. I heard the little spring make its click but didn't feel the needle go in all the way. In fact, I didn't feel it go in at all. I pushed down on the plunger, but nothing. I pushed a little harder. Still nothing.

I decided to investigate. I pulled the Quick-Serter away from my body and everything came with it. There was no needle in my stomach. I turned it over and immediately saw my problem. I had forgotten to take the blue safety cap off from around the needle and was trying to jam the whole thing into my stomach. Oops.

I remember that Bo had made this same mistake the very first time we tried injecting insertion sites at the PADRE teen retreat. He almost *punched* the plunger down, not wanting to look stupid in front of me. I made fun of him for the rest of the weekend.

Tip: Remove blue cover from infusion needle before inserting. Doh!

DAY 23 TUESDAY JANUARY 14

Spike: Three days go by so fast when you are pumping . . . I pulled out my old site, refilled my reservoir, got all set up, took a couple of breaths, and pushed the release on the Quick-Serter to inject the cannula (on the right side of my tummy this time).

Nothing happened. I heard a little click but didn't feel anything. Was I already so used to it that I didn't feel it at all?

I pushed on the plunger and the thing wouldn't budge. Hmmm? I carefully pulled the whole setup away from my body and turned it over. Sure enough, I had forgotten to remove the blue safety cap yet again. Double Doh! I hope Bo doesn't read this.

DAY 27 SATURDAY JANUARY 18: NEW BATTERY

Spike: I was sitting at my computer, playing some online chess (What? Vanessa thinks online chess is cool.) when my pump made one of those beeps. It sounded like it does sometimes on the morning I am supposed to change my insertion site. When the reservoir is low, it gives a little beep, letting me know I need to fill another one soon. It also makes the sound when delivery has stopped because of a kink in the tubing. This time I had a new message, "Low Battery."

I had had the same battery in for almost a month and now it was time for a new one. I opened my diabetes drawer (no longer full of needles, it now contains reservoirs, infusion sets, my Quick-Serter, and a bunch of AAA batteries) and took out a battery. I unscrewed the battery cover with a nickel (a dime would do or even a screwdriver, I suppose) and the old battery popped up. I stuck the new one in (being sure to put it in the same way as the old one), screwed the top back on, reactivated my pump, and was back to normal.

I hit the ESC key to check on my battery status. Sure enough it said "Battery: Normal." Woo hoo! I had mastered yet another pump skill. I am *invincible*!

Changing batteries

Bo: Carry a spare battery. When I received my pump in the mail, I put in the battery and played with it for a week before Spike and I went to see our diabetes educator. I hit every button in every possible combination just to see all the cool things it could do. When it came time to wear the pump, my diabetes educator told me I would have about a month of battery life. Of course she didn't know that I had been playing with mine for a week. A few days later, my battery died at 2:00 AM, and I had to drive across two towns to find a store that was open, so I could buy a new triple-A battery.

The battery you install has to be a brand-new, never-been-used battery. This is a safety precaution built into the pump. Along the same lines, don't install your battery upside down. This may drain the slightest bit of energy out of the battery, so that when you install it right side up, the pump thinks it's a used battery and won't accept it.

Tip: Have a stash of batteries for your pump and meter in your spare kit.

DAY 32 THURSDAY JANUARY 23

One Month on the Pump

Bo: I have discovered that being on the pump allows me freedom that I never had before. I can sleep in without worrying about my sugar. I can eat cookies when I receive them as a gift. If I get full from eating a big meal and later on my sugars begin dropping a little bit, I don't have to eat. All I have to do is lower my temporary basal. I don't have to try to stuff in more food.

I am also very happy to see that I am using a lot less insulin every day. On injections I used 75 units a day. Now, on the pump, it's more like 45 units a day. One month has gone by, and there are no regrets from this new pumper.

Spike: I am amazed at how much better my numbers have been since going on the pump one month ago. I wake up between 80 and 100 every morning (which used to be my most unpredictable time of day). And after one month, I don't even notice that my pump's there anymore.

When I was on injections, I took between 50 and 55 units of insulin each day (9–10 R per meal, 3× a day; 15 U at breakfast; 10 U twelve hours later). On the pump, I am taking 36–40 units each day.

I've also noticed that with the pump I test more often than I used to. It's more practical to test all the time, because now when I see my test results, I can do more about it. I can dial in small doses to fine-tune highs or lower my basals if I expect my sugars to drop. I used to be very skeptical about going on the pump, but now I recommend it whole-heartedly.

Tip: Most people find that when they go on the pump, they use less insulin. On less insulin, you don't have such big ups and downs, and it's healthier to use the actual amount of insulin your body needs.

Tip: Insulin is a hormone that stores fat. It is common to lose a little weight when you go on the pump. On the other hand, some people gain weight when they go on the pump, since it is easier to eat whatever you want so they go hog wild.

DAY 48 SATURDAY FEBRUARY 8

Surfing

Spike: I woke up at the crack of dawn this morning, 9:55 AM. By 10 o'clock, three of my friends had arrived and were honking the horn out in my driveway. By 10:05, I was running out my front door with my board under my right arm and a bag full of wetsuits and food in my left hand. My friends were still honking, and I think my neighbors were starting to get a little irked.

I tested my blood on the way to the beach. I was 95. Not too shabby. I have been waking up with *superb* numbers every morning since I went on the pump. Ninety-five was a little low for exercising, so I took a little less insulin for my breakfast than usual. Breakfast was a 48-carb bagel with cream cheese and a medium sized, 18-carbs or so, banana. Normally I would bolus just over 5 units for 66 carbs, but I only took 3.8. Since that was about 1.5 units less than the carbs called for, I figured my blood sugar would come up about 60 points, to 155. I tested again at the beach—this being my first time surfing since going on the pump, I really wanted to make sure I didn't get low out in the water. I was 150. I ate half a granola bar just to be on the safe side. I thought this might cause me to go high and decided not to stay out in the water for much more than an hour.

I disconnected my pump and put it in my bag in the shade. I put my wetsuit on a little more carefully than normal and made sure not to let it drag against my infusion site. I had an extra reservoir and infusion site in my bag, just in case, but didn't want to go through the hassle of inserting it again. Plus I figured that, as long as I set this up right, I shouldn't have to.

The surf was sub par and the rides were so-so. I am happy to report, however, that I didn't even notice my infusion site at all. I thought it might hurt or tear out since I was rubbing it against my board through my wetsuit, but I honestly didn't feel it one bit.

I got out of the water about an hour and a half after going in. I wanted to get out and check my sugar. Before this surf trip, I had never gone disconnected from my pump for more than 10 minutes, and I wanted to make sure I wasn't getting super high. I tested and was 90. I'm glad I had that extra bit of food before going out.

I didn't go back out in the water since the surf was so crummy. If I had wanted to, though, I think I would have eaten a bunch and taken a tiny bit of insulin. I would have needed to raise my blood sugar before going out in the water, but it is important not to go too long without any insulin at all. But since

I *didn't* go back out, I just plugged back in and had a tiny snack of crackers.

Tip: Test before you surf. Test often during an all day surf session.

Tip: Take Gatorade and plenty of snacks to the beach.

DAY 49 SUNDAY FEBRUARY 9

Fraternity Formal

Bo: Last night I attended a semi-formal dance put on by my fraternity. Dressing up was pretty easy with the pump. I used 42-inch tubing. I like using the longer tubing because it can go from the site on my stomach, below my tucked-in shirt, and come back up and into my pocket. I went to the formal with my pump in my pocket and carried my small testing kit. I use the FreeStyle tracking system, so my test kit is small—just my Palm Pilot and tester.

When the hors d'oeuvres came around, it was "a piece of cake." Bolusing for the carbs was a breeze. I had a few won tons, figured the carbs, and just dialed it in. In the past, on injections, I used to take two kits in one bag, my test kit and my insulin kit. Then when I needed to inject, I'd have to pull my shirt up and inject. Sometimes I'd just inject through my shirt. But I didn't like to do that with a dress shirt, as sometimes there would be a little blood. Injections didn't really interfere with my social life, but compared to the pump, they were a bit of a hassle. As I have discovered, you can take the pump anywhere.

Dating

Bo: When you are dating, keep in mind that being close can be exciting and very emotional, and that takes energy. The excitement of going on a date, kissing, or being close can lower your blood sugar. Before going out on a date, I test my blood sugar. If it's in my target range (80–140), I take Gatorade along to sip. If I am low, I eat some carbs and drink some Gatorade. If I have high blood sugar, I take 1/3 to 1/2 my regular correction bolus. Just the anticipation and excitement of being with your girlfriend or boyfriend can bring your blood sugar down. It's worth noting that for some young people excitement (stress) causes a rise in the hormone cortisol and a rise in blood sugar. You will figure out which way excitement sends your blood sugar.

Girlfriends and boyfriends

Bo: It is crucial that the people you spend the most time with on a day-to-day basis know everything there is to know about your diabetes. This may be your parents and siblings, your group of friends, or your girlfriend or boyfriend.

It's important to let your closest friends know about highs and lows and about your insulin routine. What you do every day to take care of yourself is part of who you are. Letting your friends in on it not only helps you, but it empowers them, and they'll feel good about helping you out should you need it.

Continuous Blood Glucose Monitor

Six months later

Bo: The continuous glucose monitoring system, known around the MiniMed site as the CGMS, is a new innovative way of monitoring glucose levels. The CGMS isn't like your regular "finger-pricking" blood testing device. Rather than only test your blood glucose levels five or six times a day, the CGMS reads your glucose levels every five minutes, continuously for three days.

When I worked at MiniMed the summer of 2003, I jumped at the opportunity to wear a CGMS. I was really excited when I finally got to put it on. The process of wearing one is almost exactly the same as inserting a pump infusion site. The CGMS has a cannula, like the one on the pump that delivers insulin, except the one on the CGMS has a sensor on the end that monitors your blood sugar levels. The sensor is about as long as the cannula on an insulin infusion site and the insertion works much the same. You put the sensor in an inserter, take off the backing on the tape so that it will stick to your site (I chose to use my stomach area—on the other side of my stomach from my pump site.) Is it painful? Well, is an insulin pump painful? NO. But to be completely honest, it was a little more awkward for me the first time I wore it (maybe just because it was new to me), because the sensor is a little stiffer than the cannula of the insulin pump infusion site. But let me tell you IT WAS AND IS AN AWESOME EXPERIENCE.

It was really cool to be able to see my blood sugars changing in real time. Now the medical professionals will say that it isn't supposed to be used to read your real time blood sugar and that only your doctor can read your blood sugars with the appropriate software, but that's not completely true. The numbers that the CGMS reads out are a measurement of voltage differences, i.e., if you have higher blood sugar it will read a higher voltage. So naturally I used my regular testing device to find out what voltage matched up with what blood sugar. When I tested, my blood sugar was 120 and the reading on the CGMS was 30. So if I wanted to know what my blood sugar was I just multiplied the reading on the sensor by 4 to get my blood sugar (120/30 = 4). This didn't replace my 6 blood tests a day, but it sure was nice to see how my blood glucose levels reacted to certain things like food, exercise, and stress (although I am so level-headed I never get stressed out!).

The three days on the CGMS was an excellent experience. I learned a lot about my body and how to better control my blood sugars, and most importantly, I was able to see trends in my blood sugars. The major shortfall of blood tests is that you only see where your sugars are at for 5 or 6 points in a day. But the CGMS gives you hundreds of points per day and gives you an overall trend. For instance, I never knew I got high blood sugar at 3:00 AM and lows at 6:00 AM (who wakes up in time to test at 6:00 AM?). But when you're wearing the CGMS it is continually "testing" your blood, allowing you to make adjustments to fix problems you didn't even know you had.

The CGMS is a great tool that everyone should try. Although I don't see myself wearing it all day, every day, I would definitely wear it before going on the pump, after I had been really sick and couldn't control my sugars, or anytime I needed to adjust my basal rates or dosing factors. It is really easy to wear and provides a lot of good information.

DAY 57 MONDAY FEBRUARY 3

Traveling

Spike: Monday was the first actual day of my new job. It was also the first time I've flown since going on the pump. I didn't think that flying with the pump would be any big deal, and it wasn't. I wasn't sure, though, so I spent a little extra time packing and preparing.

In my carry-on Rollie Bag (I had to upgrade from the duffel bag to look a little more professional), I had a stash of high-carb food: granola bars, cookies, and crackers. I also had a bag of syringes in case my pump started acting up, an extra couple of sets of reservoirs and infusion sites, and a letter from my doctor saying I was a diabetic and needed needles and pumps and all that fun stuff for medical reasons.

I have been traveling by plane weekly now, passing through security with my pump. Security has you take everything out of your pockets: your wallet, your keys, your beeper, and they even have you take off your shoes. I leave my pump in my pocket.

On this flight, one of the airport screeners pointed to the pump clip on the outside of my pocket. I told him it was plastic and wouldn't beep and sure enough it didn't. I wasn't really sure if I would beep or not, so I was pretty happy that I didn't.

Since then I have flown about a dozen times and have still never beeped. I have had a couple other screeners point out my "beeper." One lady insisted I remove it, and I pulled it out, showing her the tubing, and started to tell her what it was when she interrupted, "Oh, that's a pump isn't it? Go on through."

Tip: Carry your test kit and your spare kit, an extra bottle of fast-acting insulin, and your glucagon kit. Remember to carry these important supplies on your person. Don't check them.

Tip: When I plan to be gone for a week, I take extra batteries and insulin, a glucagon kit, ketone strips, and enough insertion sites for two weeks.

Tip: Carry the box your insulin comes in with the pharmaceutical label attached; same goes for syringes, carry the prescription label for them.

Tip: Wear your medical ID bracelet or necklace (you might have to take this off to get through the metal detector).

Tip: Carry a letter from your doctor stating you have diabetes and require insulin, syringes, and an insulin pump.

Out with the old, in with the new

Bo: Using the pump changes a lot of things, including what's in your kit. Our old kit was big and bulky: it held two kinds of insulin, an ice pack, lots of syringes, and an entire testing kit inside. The new kit is only a testing kit. Why? Because all you need in the kit that you always have with you is a way to test your blood sugar. All of your insulin and your "syringe needs" are taken care of with your pump.

New kit contains:

- Test kit

Back-up supplies need to be in your Spare Kit in case your pump breaks or malfunctions:

- A few syringes
- Bottles of insulin, fast- and long-acting
- Ketone test strips

The spare kit

My spare kit is the kit that I need when I want to change my infusion site, or when I have a problem with my pump. I keep my spare kit in my car if I am not at home, or in my Diabetes Drawer at my apartment. It doesn't really have to be easily accessible because you should only have to get to it every 3 days when you change your site or if your pump malfunctions.

Spare kit contains:

- Extra reservoirs
- Extra infusion sets
- An infusion set inserter
- IV prep swabs
- Extra batteries for your pump
- Ketone test strips
- Uni-solve swabs to remove tape gum
- Back-up supplies of syringes, bottles of insulin, and ketone test strips

The Cooler

To make life easier and more organized, you need a cooler packed with back-up food—even when you're on the pump. It should have short-, medium-, and long-lasting foods to help you treat lows in case you are away from any other source of food. It should have Gatorade or juice, granola bars, frosting or glucose tablets or gel, crackers, jerky, and a copy of *Symptoms* taped to the inside of the cooler (page 250). This is also a good place to keep a bottle of ketone test strips.

High Blood Sugar

Spike: High blood sugars happen. I often have sugars over 280 when I don't bolus enough for a meal. I test after I eat—if it turns out I am high, I bolus and test again in an hour or two, and I am fine.

If there is a clear reason for a high blood sugar—say you forgot to bolus, you miscalculated the carbs in a meal, or you ate an extra piece of pizza or a candy bar—take a correction bolus. Then recheck your blood sugar in one hour to make sure insulin is being delivered.

If there is no clear reason for the high blood sugar—check your pump, the tubing, and the site for problems. Check for ketones. If your pump checks out, and it is working correctly, and ketones are negative, take your correction bolus. Then recheck your blood sugar in one hour to make sure insulin is being delivered.

High blood sugar with ketones

Bo: Okay, now this is the important stuff: There are two reasons pumpers need to pay attention to high blood sugar with ketones. The first is that high blood sugar with ketones can set in fast when you are on the pump. Pumps only use short-acting insulin, so there is no long-lasting insulin (like U, NPH or Lantus) lingering in your bloodstream to prevent ketones. The second reason is that most kids who switch from injections (using a combination of short-acting and long-acting insulin) to the pump (which only uses short-acting insulin) do not recognize the symptoms of ketoacidosis.

Any time you have **unexplained high blood sugar** or **blood sugar over 300,** you should consider an insulin delivery problem (a kink in the tubing, the cannula has slipped, or a malfunction of your pump).

Untreated, even for a few hours, ketones can develop into that nasty condition, ketoacidosis. Fast-acting insulin lasts about 3 hours in the body (3–5 hours in toddlers). If your pump poops out, you can be out of insulin in 3 hours. Because there is no long-lasting insulin in the background, your body can start producing lots of ketones in a few hours. Catching ketones early is a good reason to test 4 or more times a day (page 132).

Tip: If your blood sugar is over 300, **always** test for ketones. (For toddlers, if you see repeated numbers in the 280s, 290s, or over 300, it's time to check for ketones.)

➠ **Note:** The number one reason kids on injections go to the ER is for low blood sugar. The number one reason kids on the pump go to the ER is for ketoacidosis.

If blood sugar is over 300 and ketones are negative
Troubleshoot the pump

- Tubing
- Site
- Pump menu (Check to make sure you took your last bolus.)

If you can't find anything wrong with your pump:

- Bolus your correction dose.
- **Don't eat.**
- Drink lots of water or sugar-free liquids.
- Test in 1 hour.
- Apply the insulin used rule (page 223).

An hour after you bolus, your blood sugar should have dropped about 1/3 of what you corrected for. If you are close to that number, things are OK. Now you can eat and bolus for the carbs. **If your blood sugar has not begun to drop, you will need to inject insulin with a syringe.**

For example: If you started at 300, bolused your correction dose, and one hour later you are at 289 or 290, your blood sugar is not responding to the bolus. Take a shot with a syringe (your correction dose). Don't mess around. Detach yourself from your pump and start all over with all new stuff: tubing, site, etc.

If your blood sugar is above 280 and you have ketones (moderate to high), you need to take insulin with a syringe.

- If you show any traces of ketones, fill your syringe with your regular correction dose and give yourself a shot.
- Disconnect yourself from your set and pump.
- Start all over with new tubing and a new set and prime the pump.
- Drink water or non-sugary liquids.
- If **injecting** your correction dose of insulin, you know the insulin is in your system, so check your blood sugar 2 hours after injecting to see if your correction dose was adequate.
- Continue to check for ketones until you test negative.
- If the ketones are gone, return to your normal pump routine.

You give your regular correction dose if ketones are trace to moderate.

If ketones are large you will need to take a shot with a syringe.

When you are on the pump and you see large ketones, call your doctor or your diabetes educator. Your diabetes team will help you figure the correction dose. It's a good idea to discuss this with them before you have high ketones.

- Fill your syringe with your correction dose. Inject.
- Disconnect yourself from your set and pump.
- Drink, drink, and drink some more water or non-sugar fluids.
- Test again in 2 hours.
- Continue to test for ketones until you test negative.
- Ketones should be going down and blood sugar should be getting back to normal.
- **If ketones still show large, call your doctor.**

The Emergency Room

Call your doctor when:

- You see large ketones.
- You can't drink fluids.
- You have vomited more than three times.
- You are feeling confused or have slurred speech.

Tip: Test, then call your doctor with your numbers written down.

Go to the ER when:

- You have difficulty breathing.
- You are unable to tolerate fluids.
- You have ketones and you are vomiting or feel really bad, like you are going to collapse.

At the ER, they can put you on IV fluids, adjust your insulin, wash out the ketones, and send you home in a couple of hours. If you wait too long, you may end up in the intensive care unit (ICU) for a couple of days.

You and your family are the experts on your diabetes. If you should go to the ER to be treated for ketoacidosis ask your parents to:

- Monitor your treatment.
- Ask the ER doctors to call your endocrinologist.
- Remind the ER doctors about your insulin pump.
- Give the hospital staff a list of your basal rates.

One Year later: Spike's airport adventure

I fly out of San Francisco weekly now with my job. As always they ask me to remove my pager before going through the metal detector. "Watch this," I say and walk through. Sure enough, no beep. The guy looks at me, puzzled. I lift my shirt to show him what it is and before I can say, "pump" he says "Oh, insulin pump, gotcha." They almost all know about insulin pumps now, but this guy was fast in catching it.

I'm about to tell him that he's the best TSA guy yet, when the guy checking the bag going through the machine says, "I'm still doing it the old fashioned way." I think he is talking about going through my bag instead of using the metal detector and look at him, quizzically.

He does the universal "injection into the hip" sign.

"No kidding?" I ask.

"Yup, how long have you had it?"

"Sixteen years next month. Since I was 7."

"Since '79." He says it with a real sense of pride. He is smiling and his buddies are smiling.

As I am putting my belt back on (I have to take it off since my giant Statue of Liberty emblazoned on the US flag belt buckle sets off the metal detector), an older TSA guy taps me on the shoulder and says, pointing across to the second metal detector, "She wears a pump." Keep in mind my flight was leaving in 10 minutes, and I was frantic and not thinking straight. I looked at him, puzzled.

"The little blond, she's got a pump."

"Oh. No kidding?" I call out to her, "You pumping too?"

She looks over at me for the first time, "Huh?"

I lift my shirt. Huge smile spreads across her face as she pulls her Paradigm out of her pocket and holds it up, just glowing.

"Dude!" I shout rather loudly, "Three diabetics at the same time. This is the best airport ever!" I get a lot of smiles from the folks with diabetes and their very supportive co-workers. The lady with the metal detector wand approaches due to all the commotion I am causing.

"What's going on?" She asks.

"You work with two diabetics! They're the best people, you know?"

"We're pretty good too, don't you think?"

"What do you mean?"

"Even those of us without diabetes are all right, right?"

"I have to disagree. Diabetics are *my* kind of people!"

She held up her wand menacingly, "If you want to get on your flight, you'd better admit that we're OK too!" The whole line of ticked-off people waiting to get past the jerk making the commotion (me) was laughing hysterically by now. Anyway, I fly out of the same gate every Sunday, so I am gonna drop off a copy of *Getting A Grip* next week. . . .

Handy Magic Formulas

Your diabetes team is going to guide you through the years. When you go on the pump, you will determine your blood sugar target range, insulin-to-carbohydrate ratio, insulin sensitivity, high blood sugar correction dose, high blood sugar with ketones correction dose, and how to treat low blood sugars. We think it is helpful to understand how the calculations that affect our diabetes care are made.

The Rule of 15 for treating low blood sugars

If blood sugar is 70 or below:

- Treat with 15 grams of fast carbs (4 oz juice or low-fat milk)
- Test blood sugar in 15 minutes

If your sugar is not above 70 after 15 minutes, drink another 15 grams of fast carbs.

- Test blood sugar in 15 minutes

When your blood sugar returns to 70 or above:

- Eat a 15-gram carb snack of longer-lasting carbs, such as crackers, and some protein and fat such as string cheese or a few nuts. This will help keep your blood sugar from dropping again.

When you treat for low blood sugar, you will not bolus for the fast-acting carbs (fruit juice or glucose tabs). You won't bolus for the longer-lasting carb snack, either. However, if you find that your blood sugar soars after the longer-lasting 15-carb snack, you can bolus for 1/2 the snack (7 carbs).

Tip: The following items have 15 grams of carbohydrate: 4 oz fruit juice, 1/2 can regular Coke or soda, 3 (5-gram) glucose tablets.

Tip: Always carry fast-acting carbs for treating low blood sugars. You should have your cooler filled with fast-acting and medium-acting carbs in your room, at school, or in your car.

Insulin-to-carbohydrate ratio

This method can be used if your pre-meal blood sugar is within your target range and your post-meal blood sugar remains below 180.

Divide insulin (bolus) taken at a meal into the number of carbohydrates eaten

$$\frac{\text{60 grams of carbohydrate eaten}}{\text{6 units of insulin}} = 10$$

Insulin-to-Carbohydrate Ratio = 1 unit of insulin to 10 grams of carbohydrate

The insulin used rule

Rapid-acting insulin (Humalog and Novolog) lasts 3 hours for teens and 90% of kids over 7 or 8 years old. It lasts 4–5 hours in toddlers and children under 7 years old. Figuring with the 3-hour rule: Blood sugar should drop 1/3 the expected amount each hour.

For example: You have a blood sugar of 340.

- Your sugar usually drops 40 points per 1 unit of insulin (insulin sensitivity).
- You would like to correct to 100.
- You need insulin to cover the 240 points above your target number of 100.
- 240 divided by 40 equals 6. Your correction dose is 6 units.

If you are a teen applying the Insulin Used Rule (3 hours), then each hour 1/3 of the insulin bolused or injected should be absorbed.

- One hour after bolus or injection of 6 units, 1/3 of the total units (2 units) should have worked.
- After one hour, your blood sugar should have dropped about 80 units and be about 260.

Two hours after bolus/injecting 6 units, 2/3 of the total units (4 units) should have worked. Your blood sugar should be approximately 180.

Tip: Insulin sensitivity is different in everybody. Your CDE will help you figure your insulin sensitivity ratio.

Correction dose

To figure your correction dose:

- Subtract your target blood sugar from your actual high blood sugar.
- Divide the answer by your correction factor to see how much insulin you need. For example: You and your diabetes team have determined that your blood sugar drops 40 points for

each 1 unit of insulin taken. Your correction ratio is 1 unit of insulin per 40 points blood sugar.
- Your target range is 80–140.
- You have a blood sugar of 240.
- 240 is 100 points above your target range.
- Divide 100 by 40. Your correction dose is 2.5 units.

Remember to use the Insulin Used Rule when figuring a correction dose within 3 hours of taking a bolus.

Correction dose: high blood sugar with ketones

Bo: I am interested in biotechnology and studying biomedical engineering in college, so the following technical approach to treating high blood sugar with ketones appeals to me. When I'm trying to figure out how much insulin to cover high blood sugar with ketones, I use my correction dose (1:40 or 1 unit for every 40 points of blood sugar I want to come down), or I use one-tenth (0.1) unit of insulin per kilo that I weigh—**whichever number is larger.**

A kilo equals about 2.2 pounds. I weigh 160 pounds, so I divide 160 by 2.2, which is approximately 70. Then I multiply 70 by 0.1 units of insulin.

$$\frac{160}{2.2} = \text{about } 70 \qquad 70 \times 0.1 = 7 \text{ units of insulin}$$

Seven units is higher than my correction dose of 5 units, so I would treat the ketones by injecting 7 units of insulin.

So, if my blood sugar was 300 and I was showing large ketones, I would figure my normal adjustment dose of 5 units to reach my target blood sugar of 100. I would also figure 0.1 unit per kilo, which for me is 7 units. I would then inject the higher number, or 7 units. If I still have ketones after injecting insulin,

I continue to test my urine for ketones every time I go to the bathroom. I drink as many glasses of water or sugar-free fluids as I can, and then I drink another glass.

Tip: If you don't have a bottle of fast-acting insulin handy, you can fill your syringe by sticking the needle into the top of the reservoir in your pump, but disconnect first.

Tip: NEVER remove the reservoir from your pump without detaching yourself from your pump first. Otherwise you may accidentally give yourself a *whole bunch* of insulin.

Tip: Talk to your doctor or CDE **now,** and write down your plan for treating ketones.

Tip: You may require 25% more than your regular correction dose if ketones are moderate to large.

Tip: Figure out how many kilos you weigh **now.** Write it down on your glucagon instruction sheet. (1 kilo equals 2.2 pounds.)

A1C and blood sugar levels

The A1C number is your average blood sugar level for the last 2–3 months. Here is a chart showing how the A1C may relate to your daily blood sugars. (Lab results may vary. Check with the lab you use for their A1C/average blood sugar correlations.)

The plus side of being on the pump

The most dramatic change is that you can skip meals. You are not constantly chasing the insulin in your system, so eating becomes a spontaneous activity.

A1C%	Average Blood Sugar
12	345
11	310
10	275
9	240
8	205
7	170
6	135
5	100
4	65

- The pump allows you to eat when you want to eat, what you want to eat, and how much you want to eat.
- You can lead a more flexible lifestyle. You can eat, sleep, exercise, etc., whenever you'd like.
- There is less chance of a super-low blood sugar.
- The pump is a conversation starter and friendship maker. People think pumpers are extremely intelligent and cool—especially if you have a good attitude about it.
- You can look up your insulin history anytime on your pump, to double-check when you last bolused for a snack or a meal.
- Pumpers usually see a decrease in their A1Cs.
- You always know the time.

The minus side of being on the pump

Bo: I spent a lot of time thinking about what my girlfriend would think about the pump, so we talked about it. She was all for it. It turns out that the pump just becomes part of your routine and when it's detached, the site is really inconspicuous, about the size of a silver dollar.

- Every once in a while the pump will say NO DELIVERY, which means the bolus wasn't delivered. To fix this I detach my pump site and reattach it. This usually works.
- It takes time to learn a new diabetes regimen.
- You will have to learn to count carbohydrates, but it's not hard.
- There is a greater chance of ketoacidosis.
- Some kids wonder whether they will be comfortable having a pump attached to them. Everyone we have talked to gets used to this very quickly.

Collected Tips

Tip: Remove blue cover from infusion needle before inserting. (Especially you, Spike.)

Tip: Don't bend over before you remove the needle. (We learned this when Spike did it.)

Tip: If your site hurts or is really uncomfortable, remove the insertion site and start over again.

Tip: You can look up your bolus history. This helps if you forget how much insulin you took and when you took it last.

Tip: Double click to make sure you bolus.

Tip: Check your pump screen right after a battery change. If it's not normal, you may have put the battery in wrong.

Tip: Make your own carb-counting sheet for everything you eat the first week.

Tip: When traveling, even if you only plan to be away for a day or two, take back-up supplies. Sets can pull out. Also, you can change your mind and stay an extra day.

Tip: Make sure your parents know how to operate your pump, so they can help if you need hospitalization for surgery, an accident, an illness, or DKA (diabetic ketoacidosis).

Tip: Become best friends with your pump manufacturer's area representative.

Tip: Safety tip for toddlers and the pump. The new Paradigm 512 and 712 pumps have safety clips with locks that hold the insulin reservoir in place—an excellent choice for toddlers because of that feature.

Tip: **Write down your basal rates.** Sometimes the pump memory erases, and over time you might forget your basal rates. Then you have to figure it out again. If your basal rates are written down, you can just reprogram.

Tip: **Never, never take your insulin reservoir out of your pump without first disconnecting the pump from your body.** The plunger on the reservoir could be accidentally pushed, giving you an overdose of insulin.

Tips for girls

Tip: Periods sometimes require higher basal rates (temp basals). *–Mary Costello, age 21*

Tip: If you want your tummy to show, a good pump site is the top of the hip or outside of the thigh.
–Anita Kaura, age 17

Tip: A good place to hide your pump when wearing tight-fitting fancy clothes is between your cleavage. Or if you're wearing an evening dress, you can put your pump on a garter belt on your leg. *–Mary Costello, age 21*

Tip: Chickster is an awesome product made by the makeup company Benefit. It's a garter that fits most insulin pumps perfectly—it's cute, is sexy, and it holds my pump against my leg better than any product I've tried that was made specifically for insulin pumps. www.benefitcosmetics.com *–Mary Costello, age 21*

Tips for Friends

Tip: Give emergency instructions to others.

Tip: Teach your friends and roommates how to give you glucose gel, frosting, or sugar when you are low, whether you are conscious or unconscious. This is a very effective treatment and usually brings your sugar up.

Tip: Teach your friends and roommates how to give a glucagon injection (page 253).

Tip: Tell your friends how to suspend or disconnect your pump. In an emergency, if you are unable to respond, they can detach your pump at the insertion site on your stomach; or they can pull the set off your skin; or they can cut the tubing, then call 911. Remember to reconnect!

➠ **Note:** I don't tell people to press Suspend because I don't want anyone to press the wrong buttons and either give me insulin or change my settings without my knowledge. This way, I will also be aware of the pump's disconnection once my blood sugar has normalized. If it was on Suspend, I might not realize it and end up high because I didn't press Resume once I was ready for insulin again. *–Mary Costello, age 21*

Tip: Learn how to suspend your pump. To suspend the MiniMed Paradigm Pump, hit the ACT button, then arrow down once to Suspend and hit ACT twice.

Tip: Post a copy of *Symptoms* (page 250) in your room. Show it to your roommates.

Tip: Post *Glucagon Instructions* (page 253) on the closet door in your room, and show your roommates how to inject glucagon.

Common mistakes

Bo: These are some of the mistakes we either heard about or made ourselves during the first few days with our pumps.

- When you do an easy bolus on the MiniMed Paradigm pump, you have to hit ACT twice. I only hit it once, so the insulin never got delivered, and I ended up having a really high blood sugar—what a drag.
- When you insert the infusion site, the directions say you should stand up, and you should. Don't sit down before you take out the needle because that hurts. (Ask my brother, he did it.)
- Don't take a shower, a bath, or go swimming for about an hour after changing your site. You have to give the adhesive on your patch time to dry.
- When your pump warns you the battery is low, change it! Avoid runs to a 24-hour convenience store in the middle of the night; carry a spare battery.

Bo answers frequently asked questions

How often should you call your diabetes educator the first month?

Call your CDE at least every week, or more often if you feel it is necessary. Never hesitate to call. They are the experts. They want to help you succeed.

How do you keep your records? in books? on a computer? do you download your meter? Palm Pilot?
I keep all of my records on a Palm Pilot.

How do you remember what day to change your infusion site?
I use up a full canister, 180 units, in three days. When I check to see how much insulin I have left, if it is low, I know I am on the third day. (One e-mailer recommended changing the infusion site on every calendar day that can be divided by 3.)

How do you get the residue of sticky tape off your stomach?
I change my site in the morning, so when I take it off, I hop in the shower with no infusion site at all. Then I am able to scrub like crazy. Soap and water are recommended. If there is still goo left on your stomach, you can wipe it off with Uni-solve swabs. Alcohol takes it off too.

What do you carry with you all the time?
I carry my testing kit in my hand, my pump on my body, a candy bar, and Gatorade in my backpack.

What do you take on trips for back-up?
Extra pump supplies: I always take enough insulin, infusion sites, and reservoirs to cover staying 50% longer than I had planned. So, for a 10-day trip I would pack for 15 days. I also carry needles and fast- and long-acting insulin, in case my pump malfunctions, and ketone strips.

Do you still carry a cooler everywhere?
Yes.

Do you carry granola bars in your pocket?
Always.

Do you carry Gatorade while driving?
Yes. I keep a bottle of Gatorade on the front seat. Always test your blood sugar before driving and keep food easily accessible from the driver's seat.

How do you feel about the change in lifestyle from injections to the pump?
So far so good—it's easier. I can snack more. But I am still getting used to it, it's only been 6 weeks. I used injections for 14 years.

After how many days did you decide you really liked the pump?
Five days.

How important is your doctor's role when you go on the pump?
Very important. Make sure you get along with your doctor and that you feel he or she is giving you good care.

How important is it that your CDE is available by phone?
Having a CDE who is available and who communicates well is as important if not more important than your doctor. The CDE is the one you'll get to know on a more intimate level. Our CDE is spectacular!

Why do you only eat 3 meals and no snacks the first few days on the pump?
You only eat three times a day to minimize all the extra variables that you have to take into account when determining how much insulin you need every day (basal rates and boluses).

Why don't you exercise the first three days on the pump?
You want to minimize the extra variables. See above.

Carb counting, how are you doing it?
We are learning by experience. The more you pay attention to counting the carbs in what you eat, the sooner it becomes second nature. Also, it's nice to have a booklet to refer to. If you have never had a certain food or meal before, look in your carb-counting book (we like *The Doctor's Pocket Calorie, Fat & Carbohydrate Counter* and *The Diabetes Carbohydrate and Fat Gram Guide*) for some help in making your estimate.

Spike and Bo's Carb-Counting Sheet

Things We Eat All the Time

Item	Quantity	Carbs
Bagel,1 baby	1 oz	15
Bagel, med	2 oz	25
Bagel, large	4 oz	55
Banana	1 small	15
Beans	1 cup	15
Beer	1 bottle (12 oz)	15
Lite beer	1 bottle (12 oz)	6
Bread	1 slice	15
Brownie	2 inch square	15
Cereal	1/2 cup	15
Chips, potato	15	15
Chips, tortilla	10	15
Cottage cheese	1 cup	8
Crackers	6	15
Cupcake, frosted	1	30
English muffin	1	30
Graham crackers	3 squares	15
Hamburger bun	1	30
Hotdog bun	1	30
Ice cream	1/2 cup	15
In-N-Out burger	1	40
Double/double	1	40
Fries (McDonald's)	medium	57
Macaroni	1/2 cup	15
Milk, whole	1 cup or 8 oz	11
Milk, whole	12 oz	15
Noodles	1/2 cup	15
Oatmeal	1/2 cup	15
Orange juice	1/2 cup	15
Peanut butter, Jif	2 T	7
Pie, pumpkin	1/8 pie	30

Things We Eat All the Time (*Continued*)

Item	Quantity	Carbs
Popcorn	3 cups	15
Potato, baked	small	30
Potato, mashed	1/2 cup	15
Rice	1/3 cup	15
Rice	1 cup	45
Spaghetti sauce	1/2 cup	15
Syrup, light	2 tbsp	15
Syrup, regular	1 tbsp	15
Tomato sauce	1/2 cup	5
Tortilla, corn	1-6 inch	10
Tortilla, flour	1-8 inch	20
Vanilla wafers	5	15
Snack bars		
Balance Gold - Caramel Nut Blast		22
Extend Bar (with cornstarch for slow release)		30
Glucerna Bar (with cornstarch for slow release)		24
Granola Bar - Quaker Chewy Choc Chip (always in our coolers)		21
Platinum Bar		10.5
Power Bar - Peanut butter		45
Make it really easy		
Beans	1/2 cup	15
Bread	1 slice	15
Cereal	1/2 cup	15
Milk	1 cup	10
Pasta	1/2 cup	15
Rice	1/3 cup	15

Meat, chicken, salad, and vegetables are free unless you have a giant serving.

[a] Notice that 1/3 cup of rice has 15

Tip: Check the back of the package for the Nutrition Facts of the foods you eat all the time. Then add your favorite foods to your personal carb sheet. We discovered that the flour tortillas we like have 20 grams of carb per tortilla.

Tip: When you look at a label, only use the carb count. (Sugars are already included in the total amount of carbs on the label.)

How do you estimate servings for carb counting?
It's a good idea to use measuring cups for your first few weeks. It sounds tedious, but measuring is a very powerful visual aid. After you look at 1/3 cup of rice that you have measured out, you'll remember how much 1/3 cup is. Again, nothing can substitute for experience. The more time you spend counting your carbs and measuring your food (if not actually measuring it, at least trying to estimate the size of portions in your head), the better you will be at getting accurate results.

Make your own carb-counting sheet
When we first started counting carbs, we wrote down everything we ate and the carb count. Pretty soon we had our own handy carb-counting sheet of our favorite foods. We suggest you make your own list, too.

Carb counting meals

Bo: We have done a little carb counting to help you get started. The first three days you are on the pump your CDE will want you to only eat three simple meals a day. This is because he or she is working on figuring out your own personal insulin-to-carb ratio. Everybody's sensitivity to insulin is different. It turns out that I need 1 unit of fast-acting insulin for every 10 grams of carbohydrate I eat. Spike needs 1 unit of fast-acting insulin for every 12.5 grams of carbohydrate he eats. It took several days to figure this out. (Remember, these are baseline numbers. When you add exercise, your insulin-to-carbohydrate ratio will change.)

Meal carb-counting sheet

DAY 1 (DECEMBER 23)

Breakfast

Bacon		
Eggs		
Potatoes/cheese	1/2 cup	15 carbs
Toast	1 slice	15 carbs
Whole Milk	1 cup or 8 oz	11 carbs

We served the fried potatoes, then measured a normal serving. It was 1 cup.	30 carbs
The average slice of bread is 15 carbs.	15 carbs
We poured a glass of whole milk, then measured it: **1 1/2 cups** (12 oz)	15 carbs
	60 carbs

Breakfast: 60 carbs

Spike is on a bolus ratio of 1 unit of insulin to 12.5 carbs, so he took 4.8 units of insulin. I am on a ratio of 1 unit of insulin to 10 carbs, so I took 6 units of insulin.

Lunch

Ham sandwich	2 slices bread	30 carbs
Milk	1 glass (12 oz)	15 carbs
		45 carbs

Dinner

Beef Stroganoff	1/4 cup sauce	4 carbs
Noodles	1/2 cup	15 carbs

Mushrooms		
Peas	1/2 cup	15 carbs
Green salad		
Diet drink		
		34 carbs

We served the noodles, then put the noodles back in a big glass measuring cup to see how much we were eating. We only had to do this a couple of times to get the hang of the size of our servings of noodles, rice, or whatever we were eating. In this case, a serving of noodles was 1 cup or 30 carbs.

The sauce was made with cream of mushroom soup (9 carbs per 1/2 cup) and a tiny dollop of sour cream, which we ignored.

Before we went back for seconds, this dinner worked out like this:

Noodles	30 carbs
Beef Stroganoff	4 carbs
Dinner:	34 carbs

DAY 2 (DECEMBER 24)

Two meals only, we got up late. (Pretty neat—we got up late, no problem with high sugars!) We had a whole gang of people here for the Christmas holiday, so we slept until noon and had to fight for breakfast:

Breakfast

Breakfast burritos contain:

Flour tortillas	10 inch	20 carbs each
Scrambled eggs		
Sausage		
Cheese		
Fried potatoes	1/2 cup	15 carbs

Fresh salsa		
Milk	1 cup (8 oz)	11 carbs

We didn't need to measure the fried potatoes this time; we just eyeballed what we put in the burritos, about 1/4 cup of filling. We each had 2 burritos and a glass of milk, (1 1/2cups).

Two burritos:	
2 flour tortillas	40 carbs
1/2 cup potatoes	15 carbs
1 1/2 cup (12 oz milk)	15 carbs
	70 carbs

Breakfast: 70 carbs

Dinner

Chicken		
Potatoes, boiled	1 cup	30 carbs
Lemon juice		
Peas	1/2 cup	15 carbs
		45 carbs

The chicken and potatoes were cooked in one pot. We only counted the potatoes. It was easier to measure the boiled potatoes than to estimate how much is 6 oz. The carb-counting book says 6 oz potatoes = 15 carbs or 1/2 cup potato = 15 carbs.

Potatoes, boiled	1 cup	30 carbs

We forgot to serve the peas (0 carbs there), so the actual carb count was 30 carbs.

DAY 3 (CHRISTMAS MORNING)

We had breakfast while we were looking in our stockings. Santa had been here!

Breakfast

Bacon		
Scrambled eggs		
Fried potatoes	1/2 cup	15 carbs
Toast	1 slice	15 carbs
Milk	1 1/2 cup	15 carbs
		45 carbs

Breakfast: 45 carbs

Lunch

Ham sandwiches (two slices of bread, ham, and lettuce), one small slice of applesauce bread, and water.

Bread	2 slices	30 carbs
Applesauce bread	1 slice	15 carbs
		45 carbs

Lunch: 45 carbs

Dinner

Turkey		
Ham		
Stuffing	1/3 cup	5 carbs (according to the book)
Mashed potatoes	1/2 cup	15 carbs
Gravy		
Broccoli, mushroom casserole		
Marinated cucumbers		
Green salad		
Brandied cranberries	1/4 cup	20 carbs

I had seconds on everything, but only counted the foods with carb: potatoes, stuffing, and cranberries, and added 2 carbs for the sauce in the broccoli casserole. Spike had thirds. Our stuffing was made with lots of veggies and sausage, so I figured it was more like 30 grams per cup.

Stuffing	1 cup	30 carbs
Mashed potatoes	1 cup	30 carbs
Cranberries	1/4 cup	20 carbs
Broccoli with sauce		2 carbs
		82 carbs

Dinner: 82 carbs

DAY 4 (DECEMBER 26)

By now we were off the strict three meals a day regimen. We were eating what we wanted to eat, when we wanted to eat it, and bolusing for the carbs.

Breakfast

Bacon		
Scrambled eggs		
Toast	1 slice	15 carbs
Milk	1 1/2 cups	15 carbs

Lunch

Turkey sandwich	2 slices bread	30 carbs
Best Foods Mayo		
Lettuce		
Pumpkin pie	1 slice (1/8th pie)	30 carbs

Dinner

Turkey enchiladas	1 flour tortilla	20 carbs
Cheese enchiladas	1 corn tortilla	10 carbs
Enchilada sauce		3 carbs per serving
Pea salad	1/2 cup green peas	15 carbs
Cucumbers		
Broccoli		2 carbs for sauce
Salad		
Lite Beer	12 oz	6 carbs

(check the label or the carb-counting book)

The enchiladas had turkey, cheese, olives, and onions in them. The enchilada sauce can listed 3 carbs per serving, so we added that. We didn't have much pea salad, so we only added 5 carbs for that one.

You'll learn to estimate your servings with all the practice that you get each day. Checking your blood sugar two hours after the meal will tell you how close you were to the true carb count of the meal. And this is just one of the many reasons we say that kids with diabetes are the smartest kids in the world.

CHAPTER EIGHT

Resources

It's helpful to discuss with other kids and their parents the diabetes products they use. Each system has different qualities and you have to find the ones that work best for you. Your diabetes educator knows about all the different meters and syringe sizes and the different pumps, so start by asking him or her what would work best for you and your situation.

We had lots of fun at the ADA annual convention trying out the new meters and gadgets, but if you can't get to one of those, you can check out the annual *Resource Guide* in *Diabetes Forecast* magazine. It comes out in January and lists all of the diabetes-related products from lancets and ketone strips to the newest pump along with the manufacturers' contact information. The following table lists our favorite diabetes products.

Our Favorites	
Products	**Supplies**
Cooler	***Playmate—Little Igloo*** Available at sporting goods stores for about $15.00. We keep a packed cooler in each car—even our girlfriends' cars. At college, we still carry a cooler everywhere.
Frosting (Packet)	***Cake Mate*** **decorative gel, Net Wt. 0.68 oz (19 g)** Available in all grocery stores. Each small tube contains 45 calories, and they cost $1.39 each. We buy them by the dozen and have them all over the house—in backpacks, coolers, our kits, and the glove compartments of cars. They are so cheap, you can put them everywhere, including up the sleeve of a wet suit. We like the white cake frosting.
Frosting (Tub)	We always keep a tub of ***Duncan Hines Home Style Creamy Frosting*** **(Chocolate Malt)** in the cupboard. If you keep it in the cupboard, then it's soft when you need to use it. We use it on graham crackers when we are low, and by the tablespoon when we are very low. We take it on camping trips.
Glucagon Kit	Always keep a ***Glucagon Kit*** on hand. Take it when you travel. It works like magic for very low blood sugar. It stops the action of insulin and raises blood sugar. You'll need a prescription. A kit costs about $90.00. Be sure to check the expiration date.
Glucose tabs	***Glucose tabs*** are used for relieving low blood sugar. Each tab contains 4 or 5 grams of carbohydrate. Read the label.

Our Favorites (*Continued*)

Products	Supplies
Glucose gel	***Glucose gel*** is used for treating low blood sugar. Each tube contains 24 grams of carbohydrate. (We keep candy bars and other sugary foods around to eat when we are low. We figure that if you are going to be low and you have to eat sugar, it might as well be something you like.) Available at pharmacies.
Gels (Sports)	***Power Bar Power Gel*** **(28 grams carb per pack) and *Gu* (28 grams carb per pack w/caffeine)** These work fast and taste pretty good. They cost $1.00–$2.50 each. Runners and bicycle riders like Lance Armstrong use it. Found in bicycle and running shops.
A1C Monitor	***Metrika A1C Now***. This is a great home-use monitor. This one-time-use, pager-sized device costs about $25.00 (you'll need a prescription) and gives you an A1C reading in minutes, with only a normal-sized drop of blood from a finger prick. Getting an A1C reading is important, because it gives you your blood sugar average for 3 months, which is necessary for good control. For example, if you had super high blood sugars at night that you weren't catching with your normal testing regimen, your A1C average would be high and alert you to the problem. We used to dread getting our A1Cs done, because it meant a costly trip to the lab and blood had to be drawn from our veins. The people at Metrika really seem to get it.

Our Favorites (*Continued*)

Products	Supplies
Ice Packs	The ***Refrigerant Gel Pack*** that comes with ***Medicool's DIA-PAK*** (see **Insulin Kit** below) lasts about a week. You will need to buy 3 small (3-inch x 5-inch) hard-plastic ice packs. ***Microban*** also makes an ice pack called ***LUNCH-PAK***. They are available in sporting goods stores.
Injection Device	***Inject-Ease (Palco Labs)*** This made it a lot easier to give ourselves our first shots. You drop the syringe into the rocket-ship-looking *Inject-Ease* and press a button. The device sends the needle into you fast. Then you push the plunger down to deliver the insulin. Available at pharmacies.
Insulin Kit	***Medicool's Dia-Pak*** It's big enough to hold a week's worth of syringes, three bottles of insulin, a granola bar, frosting, our meter kit, and more if need be. Contact DIA-PAK Diabetic Supply Organizer by Medicool at 1-800-433-2469. The address is Medicool, 23520 Telo Ave. Suite #6, Torrance, CA 90505. The cost of carrying kits range from $15.95 for the simplest daypack to $29.95 for the deluxe model. Medicool is featured in the *Shoppers Guide* portion of the ADA's publication, *Diabetes Forecast*.
Insulin Vial Protector	***Insure Insulin Vial Protector 2***, available through ***Medport.*** Individual vial holders cost $4.95 each. Good for travel and backpacking. Go to *www.medportinc.com* to order.

Our Favorites (*Continued*)	
Products	**Supplies**
Ketostix	***Reagent Strips for Urinalysis*** by ***Bayer***. They are available at just about any pharmacy. We buy the simple ketone-test-only strips. Some strips also show a color for blood sugar, but you are already doing blood sugar with your arm or finger prick test. It's less information to digest when you check for ketones if you use the simple ketone-only strip. A bottle of 50 costs about $12.95.
Lancet Devices (Pricker)	***TheraSense FreeStyle*** It works on the arm. Awesome. TheraSense introduced us to the idea of testing our forearms or legs, and we like the testing device they provide. Testing the forearm is painless, plus you have a much larger surface area to work with.
BD Lancet Device	If you are still testing your blood via the fingertips, we like the ***BD Lancet*** device. They last a long time and you can adjust them for depth, in case you just can't get blood out of your finger for some reason. They cost about $12.95.
Lancets	***BD Ultra Fine II*** These seem to be a little slimmer, and they feel better than others. They work with the TheraSense lancet device. A box of 200 costs from $15.00 to $17.00
MedicAlert	***MedicAlert Bracelet*** or ***Necklace*** available for $35.00. Contact MedicAlert at 1-800-432-5378, Medical ID jewelry at www.laurenshope.com

Our Favorites (*Continued*)

Products	Supplies
Meters	***OneTouch Ultra (LifeScan)*** We really like this meter. It is super-small, only uses a tiny bit of blood, and gives you a reading in just 5 seconds. If you like testing your forearm instead of your fingers, you can use a OneTouch Ultra for that too. Visit *www.lifescan.com* or call 1-800-227-8862 for more information. This meter costs about $70.00 (but sometimes different pharmacies have promotions where they give the meter away when you buy 100 strips), 100 strips cost about $75.00. ***OneTouch UltraSmart (LifeScan)*** By the time you read this, this meter will be in the stores. It will have loads of tracking and trending capabilities (like the *TheraSense Tracker* below) and gives results in just 5 seconds, like the OneTouch Ultra. We are looking forward to this meter. ***TheraSense Tracker*** We just got two of these, and they are awesome. You can keep track of all of your information so easily and see trends to help you get a better grip on your diabetes. The cost of the PDS (Personal Digital System), module, and software is about $299.00, but it comes with a $75.00 rebate. Module and software only is $149.00, with a $40.00 rebate (you would then use your own PDA, such as a HandSpring or Visor). ***TheraSense Freestyle*** If you can't afford the Tracker, or just don't feel like storing all that information all the time, we still recommend this TheraSense meter. Bo has used it for a year and

Our Favorites (*Continued*)	
Products	**Supplies**
Meters (*Continued*)	loves it. It uses very little blood, and you can take up to a minute and a half to get blood on the strip (when your fingers aren't bleeding a lot, this helps save money). The FreeStyle is available from *www.therasense.com* or 1-888-522-5226. (Our local drugstore often has specials where you get the meter free if you buy a bottle of strips.) The cost of the meter is $75.00, and it comes with a $40.00 mail-in rebate. 100 strips cost $69.95.
Snack Bars	***Extend Bar*** Good before-bed snack. Helps stabilize blood sugar for up to 9 hours. Go to www.extendbarworks.com. Four bars cost about $5.00. ***Glucerna Bar*** Tasty snack bars. Use them when playing sports. Get them at *www.glucerna.com*. Four bars cost about $6.50. ***NiteBite Bar*** Made with cornstarch. They help keep blood sugars level during the night. Good before-bed snack. ***Platinum Bars*** We met the creators of these bars at the 2002 ADA National Convention. They are good people doing research on how their bars help to keep sugars down. Go to *www.platinumperformance.com* to order. ***PowerBars and Cliff Bars*** These are packed with carbs. Lots of kids eat them when they are into heavy exercise.
Sugar Free Cookies	We discovered ***Murray Sugar-Free Shortbread and Sandwich Cookies*** at the 2002 ADA Convention in San Francisco. Tasty.

Our Favorites (*Continued*)

Products	Supplies
Syringes	Bo used ***BD Ultra Fine II*** and Spike used the ***BD Ultra Fine II Short Needle***. Bo used an injection device. He found that using the device with the short needle didn't get the needle in deep enough and hurt sometimes. Spike just injected by hand so he preferred the shorter needle.
Visual Chemstrips	We have used ***Chemstrips*** since we first got diabetes. They give you a good read, are handy when your battery goes dead, or for back-up on trips. There are 25 or 50 strips to a container. They cost about one dollar each. You can use sharp scissors to cut the strips in half right down the middle and double your money's worth. Most people use glucose meters and read their blood sugars electronically. We have found that visual Chemstrips are good for double-checking the accuracy of your meter.

Symptoms

This is what works for us. To make it yours, simply put your name in place of Bo's and list your specific symptoms. Give a copy to all your teachers, coaches, friends' parents, and close friends—basically everyone you know. And be sure you have a "Permission to Treat Document" on file at your local hospital.

When Bo Shows These Symptoms

Mild
- Headache
- Stomachache

Serious	• Feels empty • Shaky hands	• Clammy • Feels faint
Extreme	• Very upset • Tears • Disoriented	• Angry • Collapses

Do this

1. Give him some fruit drink (Gatorade) from his cooler or backpack.
2. Follow with a granola bar, crackers, and then jerky.

Your role

- These symptoms are listed in the order they usually appear. If you are with Bo while he is feeling empty and shaky, is disoriented or upset, then you need to open the juice can or Gatorade, put it into his hands and make sure he drinks it. Hand him the opened granola bar and make sure he eats it.

Why is this happening?

- These symptoms occur because his blood sugar is dangerously low. He is about to pass out. At this point his thinking is cloudy, he cannot function, and he needs sugar.

Be sure to call

- If you see the more serious symptoms after giving him a sugar drink, give him more sugar drink.
- Call his Mom or Dad.
- In about 10 minutes, follow with cookies, milk, crackers, chips, and jerky.

Tip

- Kids with extremely low blood sugar may act super-silly, listless, or even belligerent. They can't eat. Put some sugar or frosting in his mouth. He will snap out of it in 5 minutes or so. If you don't know what to do—call 911.

Extreme Emergency

If Bo should pass out

- Open the frosting (or glucose gel) in his cooler or backpack immediately.
- Squirt all of it into the corner of his mouth between his cheek and gums.
- If no frosting is available, put regular sugar in the corner of his mouth between his cheek and gums. As soon as he is alert enough to swallow, follow with a fruit drink, real Coke, or Gatorade. Call his Mom, call his Dad.
- Give a glucagon injection if available. Follow the instructions on the box.
- Call 911 or go to a hospital. Tell them he is suffering from low blood sugar, which is insulin shock, and he needs glucose.

Important phone numbers

Mom

____________________Home ____________________Work

____________________Cell

Dad

____________________Home ____________________Work

____________________Cell

Doctor

____________________Office

____________________Emergency number

Local Hospital or Emergency Room number

____________________.

Using Glucagon

Glucagon is an anti-insulin hormone. It also causes the liver to release sugar into the bloodstream. That's why, even after throwing up, or when you can't eat any food, an injection of glucagon will raise your blood sugar immediately.

Tip: If you vomit once, get your back-up team in place. Call home or alert a friend that you may need help.

When do you use glucagon?

Tell your family, friends, and housemates to inject you with glucagon if:

- You pass out.
- You can't wake up, or if you seem disoriented and don't make sense.
- You are too woozy to do anything.
- Your blood sugar is falling, and you can't keep anything down.
- Remember, if things seem out of control, it's okay to call 911!

When you get a little older, you may find yourself in a situation where you need to give yourself a glucagon shot. If you have time, tell someone you are low, and you need help. Have them there or on the phone as back-up when you use glucagon, just in case you are too fuzzy to do it.

How to use glucagon

- Inject the liquid in the syringe into the bottle of glucagon powder (or tablet).

- Shake the bottle until the glucagon dissolves and becomes clear.
- Draw all the glucagon solution into the syringe. (For kids under 45 pounds, only use 1/2 solution.)
- Inject all the solution into the leg or butt.
- Roll the person onto his side. When he wakes up, he may throw up.
- Give food as soon as he wakes up:
  - Gatorade
  - Cookies
  - Crackers
  - Anything he can eat

Tips

- Always keep a glucagon kit in your diabetes drawer or cooler.
- Check your drawer/cooler right now. Make sure your glucagon kit is up to date.
- You can use an insulin syringe for glucagon. You may have to inject twice because insulin syringes hold less.
- Fifteen minutes and again thirty minutes after a glucagon injection have a snack of juice, crackers, and protein to help keep blood sugars level.

Other Books to Read

Carb Counting Made Easy, McCarren, ADA, 2002. One of the Fast Facts series of 64-page books, includes lists of foods.

The Official Pocket Guide to Diabetic Exchanges, 2nd edition, ADA, 2003. Includes all the foods on the Exchange Lists and the carb counts.

Carbohydrate Counting—A Primer for Insulin Pump Users to Zero in on Good Control, MiniMed www.minimed.com.

The Complete Guide to Carb Counting, 2nd edition, ADA, 2004. Includes food lists with carb counts and special sections for pumpers.

Getting a Grip on Diabetes for Kids and Teens, Spike and Bo Loy, ADA, 2002. This is a how-to book for kids. We were on injections when we wrote this book. It is full of tips and techniques for handling diabetes at school, during sports, while traveling, and with your friends.

Real Life Parenting of Kids With Diabetes, Virginia Loy, ADA, 2003. A how-to book for parents, written by our mom. It is kind of like *Getting a Grip* for parents, and we all know that a lot of times parents just need to get a grip.

The Doctor's Pocket Calorie, Fat & Carbohydrate Counter, Borushek, Family Health Publications, 2003.

The Diabetes Carbohydrate and Fat Gram Guide, 3rd edition, Lea Ann Holzmeister, ADA, 2004.

Guide to Healthy Restaurant Eating, 2nd edition, Warshaw, ADA, 2002. Carb counts for more than 3,500 dishes at more than 55 chain restaurants.

The MiniMed Insulin Pump Workbook. This workbook is thorough and very clearly written. www.minimed.com

Putting Your Diabetes on the Pump, Kaufman, Halvorson, and Lohry, ADA, 2002. Another in the Fast Facts series of books. If you still haven't made up your mind about the pump, try this book.

Smart Pumping, Wolpert and Anderson, ADA, 2002.

Pumping Insulin, Walsh and Roberts, Torrey Pines, 2002.

Taking Diabetes to School, Betschart, Wiley and Sons, 1998. Great for younger kids.

Wizdom Kit, ADA. Great information and fun stuff for kids with diabetes. www.diabetes.org/wizdom

Useful Web Sites

www.benefitcosmetics.com—Chickster, garter that holds insulin pumps.

www.calvin.biochem.usyd.edu.au/GIDB/searchD3.htm—It is great if you'd like to find the glycemic index value of specific foods.

www.diabetesnet.com—An awesome place to find information and buy diabetes books and products.

www.diabetes.org—The American Diabetes Association (ADA) site with information, help, and lots of books.

www.nal.usda.gov/fnic/cgi-bin/nut-search.pl—Allows you to type in a food and find all its nutritional facts, including carbs and fiber content.

www.insulin-pumpers.org—A good site even for non-pumpers. It has amazing links and practical advice and photos. Great if you're thinking about pumping, are pumping, or are looking for great diabetes links on nutrition facts, carb counting, insulin types, and pump options.

www.pump-pouch.com—Pump pouches for kids.

www.pumpwearinc.com—Pump pouches for kids.

Index

About the American Diabetes Association

The American Diabetes Association is the nation's leading voluntary health organization supporting diabetes research, information, and advocacy. Its mission is to prevent and cure diabetes and to improve the lives of all people affected by diabetes. The American Diabetes Association is the leading publisher of comprehensive diabetes information. Its huge library of practical and authoritative books for people with diabetes covers every aspect of self-care—cooking and nutrition, fitness, weight control, medications, complications, emotional issues, and general self-care.

To order American Diabetes Association books:
Call 1-800-232-6733. Or log on to http://store.diabetes.org

To join the American Diabetes Association:
Call 1-800-806-7801. www.diabetes.org/membership

For more information about diabetes or ADA programs and services:
Call 1-800-342-2383. E-mail: AskADA@diabetes.org or log on to www.diabetes.org

To locate an ADA/NCQA Recognized Provider of quality diabetes care in your area:
www.ncqa.org/dprp/

To find an ADA Recognized Education Program in your area:
Call 1-888-232-0822. www.diabetes.org/recognition/education.asp

To join the fight to increase funding for diabetes research, end discrimination, and improve insurance coverage:
Call 1-800-342-2383. www.diabetes.org/advocacy

To find out how you can get involved with the programs in your community:
Call 1-800-342-2383. See below for program Web addresses.

- *American Diabetes Month:* Educational activities aimed at those diagnosed with diabetes—month of November. www.diabetes.org/ADM
- *American Diabetes Alert:* Annual public awareness campaign to find the undiagnosed—held the fourth Tuesday in March. www.diabetes.org/alert
- *The Diabetes Assistance & Resources Program (DAR):* diabetes awareness program targeted to the Latino community. www.diabetes.org/DAR
- *African American Program:* diabetes awareness program targeted to the African American community. www.diabetes.org/africanamerican
- *Awakening the Spirit: Pathways to Diabetes Prevention & Control:* diabetes awareness program targeted to the Native American community. www.diabetes.org/awakening

To find out about an important research project regarding type 2 diabetes:
www.diabetes.org/ada/research.asp

To obtain information on making a planned gift or charitable bequest:
Call 1-888-700-7029. www.diabetes.org/ada/plan.asp

To make a donation or memorial contribution:
Call 1-800-342-2383. www.diabetes.org/ada/cont.asp